Psychedelics for Brain Health

Psychedelics for Brain Health

Exploring The Mind-Enhancing
Potential of Psychedelics
For Cognitive Well-Being

Fred Grover Jr. M.D.

Copyrighted Material
Psychedelics for Brain Health:
Exploring The Mind-Enhancing Potential of Psychedelics
For Cognitive Well-Being

Copyright © 2025 by Fred Grover Jr. M.D.
All Rights Reserved.

No part of this publication may be reproduced, stored in a retrieval system, or transmitted, in any form or by any means—electronic, mechanical, photocopying, Recording, or otherwise—without prior written permission from the publisher, except for the inclusion of brief quotations in a review.

For information about this title or to order other books and/or electronic media, contact the author at: PsychedelicsforBrainHealth.com

Published by Spiritual Genomics Press

SPIRITUAL

GENOMICS

ISBN (Paperback) 978-1-7337722-8-0
ISBN (Amazon eBook) 978-1-7337722-9-7
ISBN (Ingram eBook) 979-8-9999894-0-6

Printed in the United States of America

Edited by Anja Brokaw
Cover Artwork by Martin Bridges

In Appreciation

With heartfelt gratitude, I thank my family, friends, and colleagues who have supported, challenged, and inspired me along my journey of growth and transformation in this lifetime, especially my parents, who have been the most loving and supportive people one could ever imagine. To my father, who committed his life with the greatest strength and love to his family and the thousands of patients he healed with his skillful open heart surgery. While he is still with us, I fear he may not recognize me within a few months of publishing this book. For that reason, I dedicate this book to him and others suffering from cognitive decline. I hope this book catalyzes more innovative solutions for those suffering from this and neurodegenerative disorders. In my daily life, I aim to make a meaningful difference in some way, so that together we can help ease human suffering. While I am here for just a nanosecond in the large perspective of this planetary age, I hope that my words and service in collaboration with others will make a positive impact now and into the future.

Contents

	In Appreciation v
	Introduction xi
Chapter 1	The Crisis of Neurodegenerative Diseases and the Potential of Psychedelics 1
Chapter 2	Enhancing Cognition, Creativity, and Problem-solving with Psychedelics 41
Chapter 3	Psychedelics for Mood Support, Anxiety, and PTSD. . . 49
Chapter 4	Microdosing Psilocybin for Enhanced Cognition and Brain Health. 63
Chapter 5	The Potential of Psychedelics to Treat Neurodegenerative Diseases 79
Chapter 6	Psychedelics Benefits to the Microbiome and the Gut-Brain Connection. 99
Chapter 7	Unlocking the Benefits of Expanded Consciousness and Awakening through Psychedelics. 103
Chapter 8	Synergistic Therapies for Brain Health 117
Chapter 9	Regenerative Medicine Therapies. 137
Chapter 10	Final Thoughts. 171
	References 177

Image References. 189

Recommended Reading 191

Recommended Websites 195

About the Author 197

About the Cover Artist,
Martin Bridges. 198

Disclaimer

The information presented in *Psychedelics for Brain Health* is for educational and informational purposes only. It is not intended to diagnose, treat, cure, or prevent any disease. The content explores emerging science and potential therapeutic applications of psychedelic substances, drawing on current research, clinical perspectives, and anecdotal experiences with plant medicines in legal local or international settings.

This book **does not** constitute medical advice or a recommendation to use psychedelics. These substances remain controlled in many jurisdictions, and use outside of approved clinical or research settings may be illegal and carries significant risks. Always consult a qualified healthcare professional before making any decisions regarding mental health treatment or psychedelic use.

If you are under the care of a psychiatrist, neurologist, therapist, or other specialist, consult with them—preferably one with expertise in psychedelics—before considering any use, to ensure a collaborative and individualized safety and risk–benefit assessment. This applies equally to those under the care of a primary care physician.

Psychedelics can pose heightened risks for individuals with certain psychiatric conditions, including schizophrenia, schizoaffective disorder, bipolar disorder (especially type I), borderline personality disorder, severe anxiety with panic attacks, depersonalization/derealization disorder, and active substance use disorders. They may also destabilize those with complex PTSD or a personal/family history of psychosis or bipolar disorder, particularly in the absence of professional screening, supervision, and integration support.

Neither the author nor the publisher assumes responsibility for any outcomes resulting from the application or misuse of the information contained in this book. Always follow local laws and regulations, and prioritize safety, legality, and professional guidance in all health-related matters.

Introduction

We are at the forefront of an exciting new era of brain health! Psychedelic medicine research is accelerating and offering great hope for the potential treatment of Alzheimer's, age-related cognitive decline, and neurodegenerative disorders. The goal of this book is to increase awareness amongst the medical community and general public about the potential cognitive benefits of psychedelics, and to stimulate novel research with plant medicines and man-made molecules. I am a Primary Care Physician, and being on the frontline of medicine for over thirty years has allowed me to see a greater diversity of medical and mental health conditions than most subspecialists. The stories and intense struggles patients have shared with me over the years have been challenging to hear and, oftentimes, difficult to address. While I am not a world-famous neuroscientist or mycologist, I offer a unique, humble perspective that I hope will help enhance the health and happiness of many. In that light, I encourage everyone also to read books recommended at the end of this book by experts, including Robin Carhart-Harris, Roland Griffiths, David Nutt, Dale Bredesen MD, Paul Stamets, and others, to go deeper in your understanding of this very complex and evolving topic of psychedelic benefits for brain health. An extensive list of references is provided as well. My goal is not only to help alleviate suffering, but also to promote happiness, well-being, and longevity.

One of my most significant concerns has been the medical community's inability to treat depression and prevent suicidality. The current pharmacotherapy utilizing traditional SSRIs, SNRIs, etc is marginally effective at best, which can lead to prolonged suffering. Looking for solutions beyond the Rx pad, I began a personal exploration of psychedelics for myself and the potential benefits for my patients. My journey began after suffering from a major depression following the tragic death of one of my best friends. I sought help, and a psychiatrist prescribed an SSRI and sent me out the door in 10 minutes with a smile, saying, "This will resolve your grief and depression." It offered nothing other than a blunting of my emotions, and as a result, I discontinued it after a few months. Somewhat synchronistically, I was introduced and encouraged to join a two-year course in Peruvian Shamanism. It was during this time that I discovered the benefits of plant medicine, particularly Ayahuasca and psilocybin, which completely cleared my depression. Ongoing work with plant medicines has kept me feeling balanced and happy. While some may find benefits from SSRIs, many will not.

My current perspective and passion in psychedelic medicine is derived not only from my shamanic psychedelic healing experiences, but also from witnessing the therapeutic benefits of psychedelic medicine therapy (Ketamine) in helping my patients suffering from depression and anxiety. I've seen many more patients clearing their depression and developing renewed passion, creativity, and enhanced cognition in their lives via modern psychedelics and plant medicine therapies than traditional psychiatric psychotropic medications. Many have discovered plant medicine therapy independently, and I have noted impressive outcomes in the resolution of their depression.

I could have remained 100% in the mainstream, prescribing the latest psychotropics like most of my peers. But when large meta-analyses revealed that antidepressants are, in many cases, no more effective than a placebo, and often cause emotional blunting, I decided to be more conservative and cautious when prescribing this class of medications.[1]

This holds true for the treatment of cognitive impairment as well. I can go the simple route of prescribing minimally effective placebo-level pharmacotherapy for Alzheimer's, or seek to heal them from a more integrative and functional medicine perspective.

Beyond patients complaining of depression, I often also get the question: "Doc, my memory seems to be off a bit. Am I developing Alzheimer's? If not, could it be that I'm simply getting older—and if so, how can I reclaim the memory and mental clarity I once had?"

The traditional response might be to do more crossword puzzles, learn a new language or musical instrument, and in some cases, be prescribed stimulants like Adderall (amphetamine) and Provigil (Modafinil). For more concerning moderate impairment, physicians may reach for cholinesterase inhibitors like Aricept (Donepezil), or NMDA agonists like Namenda (Memantine) in Alzheimer's cases. Again, most of these prescriptions are no better, or only slightly better than placebo, and do not reverse cognitive impairment. Most docs will refer out for formal neurological evaluation and testing as indicated, but in most cases, patients are looking at a 6-12 month waiting time to be seen.

Cognitive impairment has become a significant concern for my patients, particularly for those over 50. Some are concerned because they have a mother or father with Alzheimer's, and others are experiencing difficulty or slowness with recalling names or words. A history of traumatic brain injury (TBI) in the past from playing college sports, or more recent events such as falling off a bike while wearing a helmet, or car accidents with a coup/counter coup (whiplash) TBI are common. Some have a history of alcoholism or other medical conditions, such as sleep apnea, metabolic syndrome, or diabetes, that also raise their risk.

One of the primary reasons I'm writing this is because I had a paternal grandfather with Alzheimer's and am now witnessing my 86-year-old father in the early to mid stages of this condition.

I dread the day when he may not recognize me or other family members. Even though his physicians and I are doing all we can to help him preserve his memory from an allopathic and integrative medicine standpoint, it's just lightly tapping the brakes on his degenerating condition. Observing his providers applying allopathic therapies that offer minimal benefits at best has been difficult to witness. My father is a retired heart surgeon who often put in 100-hour work weeks, working into his late 70s, he logged many sleepless nights doing heart and lung transplants, and encountered massive amounts of stress in his life. There is no doubt that this non-stop lifestyle prematurely aged him and likely increased his risk of Alzheimer's while also accelerating the onset. At 84, he had notable mild cognitive impairment, and he was referred to neurology for further testing. Blood tests, unfortunately, displayed an elevated p-tau/Abeta ratio along with concerning findings in his cerebrospinal fluid. This and his cognitive testing, sadly, helped confirm his mostly untreatable diagnosis of Alzheimer's. His father also succumbed to Alzheimer's in his mid-80s, so family history is a clear risk factor too. Watching my loving father, a brilliant world-famous heart surgeon, decline has been disheartening. Why can't we do more for him and the millions of others suffering from this condition? As a family doctor providing a functional-medicine approach, I'm looking way outside the box to offer him therapies that show promise without causing harm. Even though my genetic tests (no copies of APOE ε4) do not put me at an increased risk for Alzheimer's, we are all at risk. My goal is to find innovative ways to keep all of us sharp, happy, and functional into our 90s and beyond!

In my practice, I focus on prevention, wellness, and regenerative medicine. Yes, I also take care of acute and chronic medical problems, but these become less common when a practice focuses on wellness, rather than sick care medicine. Helping my patients maintain a healthy and sharp mind is naturally one of my top priorities.

Decades of practicing medicine on the frontline and thousands of encounters have given me ample exposure to witness longitudinal cognitive decline in many of my patients. While I am not a neurologist, I am the first to encounter patients and address their issues before they are referred for additional confirmatory diagnostics and treatment by specialists. Early diagnostic blood and imaging tests with improved accuracy are now available, but they remain expensive with spotty coverage by insurance. Until we can test more affordably and with enhanced accuracy, early intervention will be limited.

We must be more open-minded, curious, and willing to explore all options, including integrative medicine therapies such as transcranial near-infrared light therapy, mitochondrial optimization (NAD+, methylene blue), nutrition, hormone optimization, neurofeedback, exercise, mindfulness-based strategies, sound healing, and, of course, psychedelics. I wouldn't be as open-minded and creative as I am today without having personally benefited from psychedelics.

As I strap on my highest-lumen hiking headlamp, I set out to illuminate the vast and intricate terrain of psychedelics for brain health, casting the brightest, most expansive light possible on this evolving frontier in the chapters ahead. This will be an evolving manuscript with future editions to come as we are enlightened further in this ongoing renaissance of psychedelic medicine. I invite you to don your headlamp as well - to explore this path with curiosity and clarity. But when the moment calls, switch off the light, lie beneath the stars, breathe deeply, and journey inward, whether through meditation or your favorite psychedelic. Envision a new future for humanity - one illuminated not just by science, but by the wisdom of your inner cosmos and ancient shamanic healers before us. Dream of a new future for humanity. One of unity, love, and collectively healing and sustaining one another.

Let the journey begin…

CHAPTER 1

The Crisis of Neurodegenerative Diseases and the Potential of Psychedelics

Alzheimer's risk and the costs of treating it are increasing at an alarming rate. In 2025, approximately 7 million people aged 65 or older suffer from Alzheimer's, by 2060 this is projected to rise to 14 million.[1] According to the 2025 Alzheimer's Disease Facts and Figure report, by 2050 the number of annual new cases of Alzheimer's and other dementias is expected to double.[2]

Let's dive more into the statistics and explore the current data of Alzheimer's risk.

Your current lifetime risk of developing Alzheimer's depends on factors such as age, gender, family history, and genetics.[3] Here's a general breakdown:

Your age-related risk
- At the age of 45, the lifetime risk is approximately 10–12%.
- At age 65, the lifetime risk increases to 10–20%.

- At the age of 85, the risk increases to approximately 33–50%.

Gender related risk
- Women: Higher lifetime risk (~1 in 5, or ~20%).
- Men: Lower lifetime risk (~1 in 10, or ~10%).
- Women live longer on average, which contributes to their increased risk.

Your risk by Family History & Genetics
- Having a first-degree relative (parent/sibling) with Alzheimer's increases the lifetime risk to 30–50%.
- APOE ε4 gene (a genetic risk factor)
- One copy of APOE ε4: ~20–30% risk
- Two copies of APOE ε4: ~50–70% risk.

How can you reduce your risk?
- A healthy lifestyle (exercise, diet, cognitive engagement) may lower risk by 30–40%. (i.e., Bredesen Protocol diet, part of his ReCODE Program - Reversal of Cognitive Decline. It and other similar diets may help slow progression, but additional larger trials are needed to confirm and demonstrate reversal of Alzheimer's with any kind of diet.) Reversing diabetes can make a significant impact on slowing disease progression and reducing the risk of developing it.

- Managing heart health (blood pressure, cholesterol, diabetes) reduces risk.

- Avoiding smoking and excessive alcohol helps protect brain function.

- Consideration of psychedelics, regenerative and functional medicine approaches to enhancing brain health.

A Quick Summary
- Average lifetime risk: ~10–20% for the general population.

- Higher for women, those with a family history, or APOE ε4 carriers.

- Modifiable lifestyle factors can significantly lower the risk. (i.e. Reverse Diabetes)

Tragically, over 500,000 Americans are diagnosed with Alzheimer's, and 120,000 die from it annually, according to the CDC.[4] Deaths from Alzheimer's and other dementias are likely grossly underreported.

The cost of Alzheimer's in 2024 for medical and long-term care was projected to reach $360 billion in the US. The impact on a family with one member afflicted is a staggering $400,000, with most families shouldering 70% of that cost.[1] So, preventing it may easily save a family $500,000 in the future. An estimated 6.7 million older adults have Alzheimer's disease in the United States. That number is expected to double by 2060.

In my opinion, the 2025 cuts to Medicaid will lead to rising rates of Alzheimer's, as thousands of diabetics are not diagnosed early and not managed proactively. Many existing diabetics also won't be able to afford medications if they are among the estimated 16 million predicted to lose health care insurance. The risk of Alzheimer's is increased by 1.5 to 2 times in Type 2 diabetics, so the short-term benefits of cutting Medicaid coverage could cost the country two to three times as much in the long term.

According to the CDC's National Health and Nutrition Examination Survey (NHANES)[5], between August 2021 and August 2023, 40.3% of adults aged 20 and above were obese (defined as a BMI of 30 or higher). This includes 39.2% of men and 41.3% of women. We will likely see half the population being obese if we don't take a much more proactive approach to this epidemic soon! According to a 2023 report in the National Center for Health Statistics, approximately 16% of our population is diabetic already. The statistics on obesity and diabetes are an ominous dark cloud shadowing our health care system and will lead to an alarming rise in Alzheimer's, neurodegenerative disease, cardiovascular disease, strokes, joint replacements, etc, over the coming decades.

Hopefully, some of the therapies I'll discuss in the following chapters will help many become aware of their unhealthy habits and trend them towards wellness, reducing the financial burden to families and our unsustainable healthcare system. I passionately feel that a healthier, happier mind through psychedelic therapies can lead to improved motivation towards a healthier lifestyle.

Future Alzheimer's Research Possibilities

While there's no silver bullet for brain health, psychedelics are part of the multi-pronged key to unlock the prevention and reversal of Alzheimer's and other forms of dementia. Harnessing the power of artificial intelligence (AI) within a more progressive, open-minded research environment will accelerate its advancement and unlock even more innovative treatment strategies. AI can also be deployed to analyze past neuroscience research data and propose new research hypotheses, along with promising interventions to consider in future trials. Finding innovative ways to go beyond monotherapy trials and exploring multi-therapy interventions within multiple arms of a study will accelerate the process. Creating and funding these multiple armed studies, as well as considering a broader range of objective markers as below, might provide more insights as well. Here is a short list of imaging, wearables, and blood tests to objectively analyze and help diagnose neurodegenerative conditions, including Alzheimer's.

- fMRI imaging
- PET (Positron Emission Tomography) Amyloid Scan
- SPECT (Single-Photon Emission Computed Tomography)
- Dynamic Functional Connectivity Analysis (Measures time-varying changes in connectivity between brain regions)
- Enhanced QEEG brain mapping
- Wearable EEG & Heart Rate Variability (HRV). Oura rings, smart watches, etc.

- AI-based speech & Linguistic analysis (can detect altered speech patterns, semantic coherence, and emotional tone)

- Smart Hearing aids with gyroscope movement and longitudinal AI analysis for gait decline

- Home or nursing home video movement analysis by AI tracking for instability

- Implantable microchips to monitor glucose, stress hormones, inflammatory markers, infection, and heart rate. Available for consumer use to broaden early detection

- Smart glasses to monitor for signs of cognitive decline

- Pupil Dilation & Eye Tracking (Can assess serotonergic activity)

- Neuroplasticity markers include serum BDNF levels (Brain-Derived Neurotrophic Factor) and synaptic protein expression

- Immunologic marker blood testing: such as Pro-inflammatory cytokines: IL-6, TNF-α, IL-1β (Psychedelics like psilocybin and LSD may reduce these cytokines, which are linked to depression and chronic stress). Also looking at Anti-inflammatory cytokines: IL-10, TGF-β. Increased levels suggest a potential immune-mediated mechanism for their antidepressant effects.

- Blood testing for Amyloid beta 42/40 ratio, ApoE genotype, Plasma p-tau181 or p-tau217, GFAP (Glial

Fibrillary Acidic Protein), NfL(Neurofilament Light Chain) and other emerging markers to find a higher specificity and sensitivity in detecting early Alzheimer's. Best to discuss blood testing with a neurologist.

The diversity of tests is growing rapidly and will help researchers and clinicians further understand the pathology, treatment, and enhance the early diagnosis of Alzheimer's and other neurodegenerative conditions. I'm also excited about the endless possibilities in wearable and implantable biotech devices. Unfortunately, many "smart-ring" companies lack the risk tolerance to provide continuous pulse oximetry monitoring, potentially leading to missed sleep apnea detections in many of us. I've had several patients with a greater than 90 (normal) pulse ox reported by rings that were found on a continuous monitor to have significant harmful drops in oxygen levels during sleep.

The Psychedelic Solution

Psychedelics' impacts on the brain vary based on their molecular structure and their interactions with neurotransmitters and receptors. These interactions lead to their characteristic effects on perception, cognition, and mood. I'll first discuss how various psychedelics are classified, then go into their numerous benefits to the brain.

Psychedelics are classified based on their mechanism of action, neurotransmitter interactions, and subjective effects. The major types of Psychedelics for Brain Health include classic, dissociative, and hybrid.

Classical Psychedelics (Serotonergic)

These include plant medicines and synthetic molecules that primarily act as 5-HT2A receptor agonists. A 5-HT2A agonist is a compound that activates the 5-HT2A serotonin receptor, a key receptor in the brain involved in perception, mood, and cognition. This receptor is the primary target of classic psychedelics like psilocybin, LSD, and DMT. These compounds mimic serotonin and activate 5-HT2A receptors, particularly in the prefrontal cortex, leading to visual and cognitive distortions. They also indirectly affect glutamate and dopamine transmission.

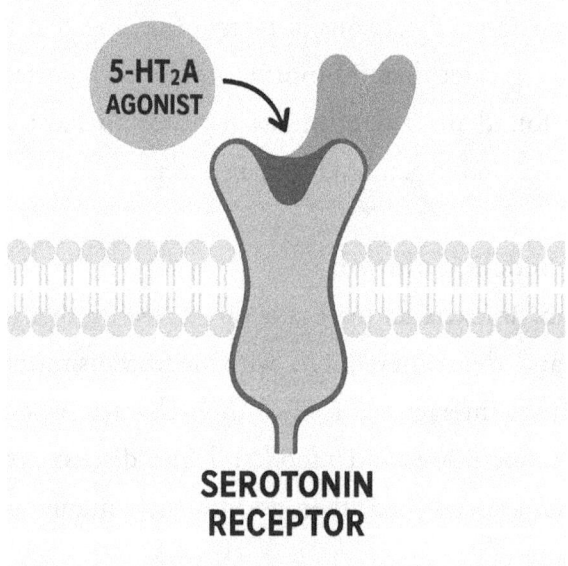

1. Interaction of 5-HT$_2$A Agonist (i.e, Psilocin) with a Serotonin receptor.

Classic Psychedelics include:
- *Tryptamines* (structurally similar to serotonin)
  - » **Psilocybin** (AKA Magic mushrooms) is the most commonly used psychedelic. Psilocybin, the psychoactive compound found in certain mushrooms, has been used for thousands of years in indigenous spiritual and healing rituals, particularly among Mesoamerican cultures such as the Aztecs and Mazatecs, who referred to it as "teonanácatl" or "flesh of the gods." After Spanish colonization, their use was suppressed, but they survived in remote regions of Mexico. In the 1950s, Western awareness was reignited when R. Gordon Wasson documented a Mazatec ceremony led by Curandera María Sabina, leading to the isolation of psilocybin by Albert Hofmann in 1958. Psilocybin research expanded during the 1960s psychedelic movement but was halted after it was classified as a Schedule I substance in 1970. In recent decades, a scientific renaissance has revived interest in psilocybin for its promising therapeutic effects on depression, anxiety, PTSD, and end-of-life distress. Psilocybin is converted to psilocin in the body, and primarily acts as a serotonin 5-HT2A receptor agonist, leading to altered perception, ego dissolution, and heightened sensory awareness. It also influences 5-HT1A receptors, which help regulate mood and anxiety. Indirectly, psilocybin modulates dopamine and norepinephrine, contributing to emotional intensity and arousal, and enhances glutamate release in the prefrontal cor-

tex, promoting neuroplasticity and expanded brain network connectivity, key to its therapeutic potential in conditions like depression, anxiety, and PTSD. A 2024 RAND Corporation survey reported that 3.1% of U.S. adults have used psilocybin during the past year.[6] That equates to approximately 8 million American adults in 2023!

» **DMT** (N,N-Dimethyltryptamine): Found in Ayahuasca, or smoked, DMT primarily affects the brain by acting as a potent serotonin 5-HT2A receptor agonist, driving its intense psychedelic effects such as vivid visuals, time distortion, and ego dissolution. It also interacts with 5-HT1A receptors, resulting in calming, anxiolytic, and antidepressant effects. It does so by inhibiting the release of further serotonin and reducing neuronal excitability. This receptor is a subtype of serotonin receptor found abundantly in the brain. Additionally, DMT influences sigma-1 receptors, which may support neuroprotection, cellular resilience, and mystical-type experiences. Though it has minimal direct action on dopamine or norepinephrine systems, DMT's rapid onset and profound effects are largely due to its potent activation of serotonergic and sigma pathways.

» **5-MeO-DMT** (Bufo Alvaris-Sonoran Desert toad venom and synthetic forms) primarily impacts the brain by acting as a potent serotonin 5-HT1A receptor agonist and, to a lesser extent, the 5-HT2A receptors. Unlike DMT, it produces less visual stimulation and instead induces intense ego dissolution, emotional release, and non-dual states of consciousness. Its high affinity for 5-HT1A contributes to its profound calming, unifying, and anxiolytic effects. 5-MeO-DMT also interacts with the sigma-1 receptor, which may play a role in its neuroprotective and consciousness-expanding properties. It has minimal impact on dopamine or norepinephrine, making its effects primarily serotonergic and deeply introspective rather than stimulant or hallucinogenic.

- *Ergolines* (Lysergamides)
    - » **LSD** (lysergic acid diethylamide), a '60s throwback, is becoming more popular and also noted for the benefits of microdosing like psilocybin. LSD is also included in the hybrid structural category of psychedelics. It impacts multiple neurotransmitter systems, primarily acting as a potent serotonin 5-HT2A receptor agonist, which drives its classic psychedelic effects like visual distortions, altered cognition, and ego dissolution. It also binds to 5-HT1A, 5-HT2C, and dopamine D2 receptors, contributing to its emotional, cognitive, and motivational effects. Additionally, LSD interacts with adrenergic receptors, which may explain its stimulating and wakefulness-enhancing properties. The 5-HT2C receptor is a serotonin receptor subtype that plays a key role in regulating mood, appetite, anxiety, and impulse control. Activation of this receptor can reduce appetite and food intake, making it a target for obesity treatments. It also modulates dopamine and norepinephrine release, affecting mood and motiva-

tion. As a result, most of us will experience a reduced appetite, happiness, and increased motivation during an LSD journey on top of the intriguing visual and sensory changes. This broad receptor activity makes LSD one of the most pharmacologically complex psychedelics, producing long-lasting and multidimensional experiences that affect mood, perception, and consciousness.

- *Phenethylamines* (structurally similar to dopamine/norepinephrine) are a diverse class of compounds that affect various neurotransmitter systems, producing effects ranging from stimulation to psychedelia and emotional enhancement. Classic psychedelic phenethylamines like mescaline (found in Peyote and San Pedro, aka Huachuma) primarily act as serotonin 5-HT2A receptor agonists, leading to visual and perceptual alterations. San Pedro is invaluable for connecting to nature and is three times longer-acting (12-14 hours) than psilocybin, making it one of my favorite plant medicines to experience in Peru.

General effects of the classics typically include visual imagery, distortions, euphoria, ego dissolution, increased emotional connection, and synesthetic experiences. A synesthetic experience with psychedelics can be a constructed, induced, or perceptual state that simulates an authentic experience. For most, LSD and pislocybin can bring in beautiful, colorful kaleidoscopic geometry. The effects are dose-dependent and vary between individuals. Enhanced brain wave activity is noted when taking these psychoactive molecules. In my view, every plant medicine or synthetic psychedelic carries its own distinct visual signature. Subtle yet profound, a plant medicine's signature can shift and evolve with each journey, making every experience uniquely personal and unpredictable. Music, in particular, can also shape-shift the ongoing imagery. In this way, psychedelics with music offer healing opportunities that can be beyond one's imagination or expectations. While setting intentions can sometimes facilitate an insight or healing, oftentimes, what is shown to you or happens is something completely different from what you envisioned. As many shamans will say, "Plant medicine will show you what you need to see." Each plant and man-made molecule has its own unique signature of effects. LSD, for example, may launch you into the cosmos with portal-like imagery similar to what you may have seen in a sci-fi movie, whereas ayahuasca brings in more earthly imagery.

Risks are possible, but fairly rare, and may include anxiety and paranoia with higher doses. Visual imagery/hallucinations are common and expected as part of the journey. These are enjoyable for most, but requires one to let go and trust in the plant medicine within a safe set and setting. Set and setting refer to the mindset (set) and environment (setting) in which a psychedelic experience occurs. Both are crucial for influencing the outcome, safety, and therapeutic value of the journey (more on this in chapter 7).

As one lets go and flows into the experience, finding healing and needed insights becomes possible. As with any psychedelic, individuals with underlying psychiatric disorders such as bipolar, schizophrenia, or severe anxiety should avoid these unless approved and used with close supervision by a psychiatrist or medical professional.

Dissociative Psychedelics

- **Ketamine:** the most well-recognized dissociative psychedelic. It's an NMDA receptor antagonist and works by blocking glutamate signaling. It often creates sensory dissociation, out-of-body experiences, "floating" sensations, altered time perception, geometric imagery, and states of oneness. These more altered states typically require higher doses. They may also offer an opportunity for a heart-opening experience, helping patients clear negative energies or traumatic experiences while often bringing in a sense of light. I've witnessed this occurring in many patients whom I have facilitated Ketamine sessions for. Integrating sound healing as part of a session can be used synergistically to potentially enhance the efficacy of psychedelic medicines.

As this molecule inhibits NMDA receptors, cortical inhibition is reduced, leading to altered consciousness and analgesic effects. You might wonder if your legs and your body are still part of you during the experience. Pursing your lips and feeling the air across them with deep breaths can help reassure and ground you.

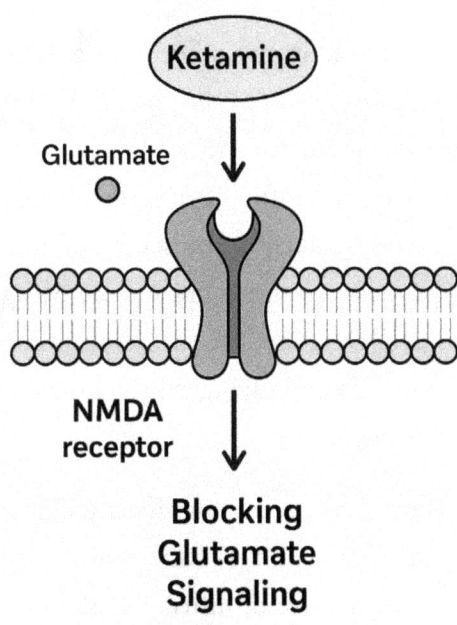

2. NMDA antagonists (i.e., Ketamine) can insert into the receptor, blocking glutamate signaling.

Ketamine also stimulates AMPA receptors, contributing to its antidepressant effects. As it enhances AMPA receptor activity, there is an increase in the AMPA-to-NMDA activity ratio believed to drive synaptogenesis and neuroplasticity. An AMPA receptor is a fast-acting excitatory glutamate receptor that helps drive learning and memory by facilitating rapid neural signaling. Ketamine was used medically for field anesthesia, particularly during the Vietnam War, and is now more often used by physicians to treat depression, and off-label to help with anxiety, OCD, and PTSD.

Ketamine is still used for anesthesia, more so in the emergency room and for short procedures.

We administer Ketamine in my office with great success for the treatment of depression, but also have a small subset of patients with depression who share how their cognition has improved after several sessions as well. After hearing this from numerous patients, my interest was piqued to study the potential mechanisms involved. Perhaps memory and cognition are being enhanced by the stimulation of BDNF and/or the resolution of depression. The deeper mechanisms underlying this phenomenon will be discussed later in this book.

Ketamine has shown rapid and significant efficacy in treating treatment-resistant depression (TRD), with response rates of 50–70% after a short course of infusions, often within hours to days. Unlike traditional antidepressants, which may take weeks to work, Ketamine acts quickly. Most studies involved IV Ketamine at 0.5 mg/kg over 40 minutes, with effects typically lasting one to two weeks after a single dose, though longer relief is seen with repeated sessions. Most providers, including myself, prefer the intramuscular (IM) dose for patients, starting at 0.5mg/Kg. We then adjust the dose based on patient response. We have seen similar efficacy with this less invasive IM route. Some providers are now using a subcutaneous fat injection, which seems to be a great option as well.

While not a cure, Ketamine can provide fast-acting relief, especially when combined with psychotherapy or maintenance strategies. However, individual response varies, and relapse is common without ongoing support or treatment. We typically recommend two sessions a week for three weeks (total of six). Patients may follow this with sublingual therapy for maintenance if they have a low risk for addiction, or they may consider doing self-administered self-administered, home-grown psilocybin microdosing.

Risks during a session may include elevated blood pressure and nausea. If significant, this can be mitigated with blood pressure and anti-nausea medication. Given the nature of this medication, you will feel sedated for a good one to two hours after a session and sometimes longer. With repeated or long-term overuse, urinary tract irritation and psychological dependence are possible. This very rarely occurs in the clinical setting and typically happens with those abusing street Ketamine. Since it has abuse potential, it should be avoided in individuals with addiction disorder and also in those with psychotic disorders. Careful screening, professional supervision, preparatory, and integration support after sessions help mitigate these risks and enhance treatment safety.

Hybrid Psychedelics (Structural and Functional)

Structural Hybrid psychedelics

These compounds combine molecular features of more than one chemical class - typically tryptamines, phenethylamines, or lysergamides - within a single molecule. Their hybrid status is based on structure, not just effects. Examples include:

- **LSD:** In addition to being considered a classic, it's also considered to be a hybrid psychedelic. Being structurally hybrid, it combines tryptamine and phenethylamine traits. Regarding its pharmacologic hybrid nature, it acts on serotonin, dopamine, and adrenergic systems. Experientially, it's a hybrid too, producing deep visuals, time distortion, cognitive shifts, and energetic stimulation.

- **2C-B:** a classic hybrid with tactile/empathogenic phenethylamine effects and mild visuals akin to LSD or psilocybin. This compound is often combined with low-dose MDMA for enhanced empathogenic impacts and has the potential to help a couple's relationship and to improve intimacy.

Functional Hybrid Psychedelics

These are substances that may belong to a single structural class but produce a blend of psychological or neurochemical effects typical of multiple drug classes (e.g., stimulant + entactogen + psychedelic). Examples include:

- **MDMA:** (3,4-Methylenedioxymethamphetamine aka Ecstasy, Molly) is primarily a serotonin-releasing agent (SRA), but has psychedelic-like effects at high doses. It's mainly appreciated for its heart-opening effects and therapeutic benefits for the treatment of PTSD. It blends properties of stimulants, entactogens, and mild psychedelics, making it a functional hybrid, though not a classic "psychedelic hybrid" like LSD. MDMA is classified as an **entactogen** or **empathogen** because of its ability to enhance emotional connection, self-reflection, and social bonding. MDMA occupies a unique therapeutic niche, often used in psychedelic-assisted therapy to facilitate emotional healing without inducing intense hallucinations or ego dissolution. It is a functional hybrid, rather than a structural hybrid. MDMA has shown high efficacy in treating PTSD, particularly in treatment-resistant cases, as demonstrated in multiple phase two and three clinical trials led by MAPS[7,8,9] (Multidisciplinary Association for Psychedelic Studies). In these trials, up to 67% of participants no longer met PTSD criteria two months after MDMA-assisted therapy, compared to about 32% in placebo groups. The benefits stem from MDMA's ability to reduce fear responses, enhance emotional processing, and increase trust and connection with therapists, allowing patients to revisit and integrate traumatic memories safely. Despite good efficacy, its approval was unfortunately blocked by the FDA in 2024 for what many consider unfounded and perhaps biased concerns. MDMA risks can include transient increases in heart rate and blood pressure, jaw tension, insomnia, anxiety, and may pose cardiovascular concerns in vulnerable individuals. An experienced and certified facilitator can help those who feel emotionally overwhelmed or anxious. Post-session integration is highly recommended. Neurotoxicity is a concern with heavy recreational use, but clinical use in controlled settings has not shown long-term harm in trials. Typically, at least a month between MDMA sessions is recommended. Post-therapy supplements such as NAC and 5-HTP are believed to help expedite recovery from fatigue on the following day.

- **Ibogaine** (Derived from the African Iboga Root) has been found to work on multiple receptors, including opioid, NMDA, and serotonin. This multimodal action makes Ibogaine one of the most pharmacologically diverse psychedelics. Its benefits have been most notably used for addiction treatment, showing potential for individuals with heroin, cocaine, alcohol, and opioid addictions. Studies and case reports suggest that Ibogaine can interrupt addiction cycles, promote psychospiritual insight, and support long-term abstinence, though results vary and large-scale randomized trials are limited. Its benefits are attributed to both neurochemical effects - modulating dopamine, serotonin, and glutamate systems - and oneirogenic (dream-like) experiences that allow deep emotional processing. However, Ibogaine carries serious risks, including cardiac arrhythmias, QT prolongation, and rare instances of sudden death, especially in those with underlying heart conditions or when used without medical supervision. Other side effects include ataxia, nausea, and psychological distress during the intense, often 12–24 hour experience, making proper screening and medical oversight essential. Thorough heart screening is vital before a session with this plant medicine. I'm excited about the future availability of Ibogaine in the United States, given its early findings and potential to treat challenging cases of addiction.

Leading ways that psychedelics support and enhance brain health:

1. **Optimizing Brain-Derived Neurotrophic (BDNF) release**

2. **Increasing neuroplasticity, synaptic plasticity, and metaplasticity** (forms of new neuron growth modulation & stronger memory connections)

3. **Activating of 5-HT2A receptors** (boosting recall & cognitive flexibility)

4. **Resetting the DMN** (Default Mode Network)

5. **Enhancing brain connectivity** (hippocampus-prefrontal cortex communication)

6. **Improving emotional memory processing** (helping with trauma & PTSD)

7. **Reducing neural inflammation**

8. **Protecting against memory decline** (potential for Alzheimer's & dementia)

Let's explore these benefits more deeply.

1. Optimizing BDNF release

BDNF is a protein (a peptide-based growth factor) that plays a crucial role in maintaining and enhancing brain health. It belongs to a family of growth factors known as neurotrophins and is often described as "fertilizer or Miracle Grow for the brain." Psychedelics are potent stimulators of BDNF, but you can also boost levels through exercise (especially HIIT), intermittent fasting and caloric restriction, Omega-3 fatty acids (esp. DHA), Curcumin, resveratrol, eating a diet high in polyphenols (such as colorful fruits and vegetables, beans, whole grains, nuts, seeds, and green tea), quality sleep, mindfulness practices, and exposure to new learning and novel experiences.

Here is a short list of psychedelics that boost BDNF, from highest to lowest based on current research[10,11].

1. **Ketamine:**

    » **Strongest and fastest BDNF surge** via **NMDA receptor antagonism.**

    » Increases **BDNF transcription and release** within **minutes to hours.**

    » **The key mechanism** behind its rapid **antidepressant effects.**

2. **LSD & Psilocybin:**

    » **Potent BDNF enhancers** through **5-HT2A receptor activation.**

    » Stimulate **neuroplasticity and synaptic growth,** but **slower than ketamine.**

    » Effects last longer but may not be as **rapid or intense.**

3. **DMT & Ayahuasca:**

    » Moderate BDNF enhancement via **serotonergic and β-carboline (MAO inhibitor) mechanisms.**

    » **Ayahuasca's harmine component** may **prolong and strengthen** neuroplastic effects.

4. **Mescaline, 2C-B, and MDMA:**

   » **Lower BDNF impact** compared to the above.

   » **Mescaline & 2C-B** stimulate 5-HT2A, but there is **less neuroplasticity research** available.

   » **MDMA has mixed results**, with some studies showing **neurotoxicity at high doses**.

Conclusion:

- If you want the highest and fastest BDNF boost, Ketamine is number one.

- If you prefer a long-lasting neuroplasticity effect, LSD/psilocybin are strong choices.

- If you want a natural source with potential sustained benefits, Ayahuasca (harmine + DMT) may help.

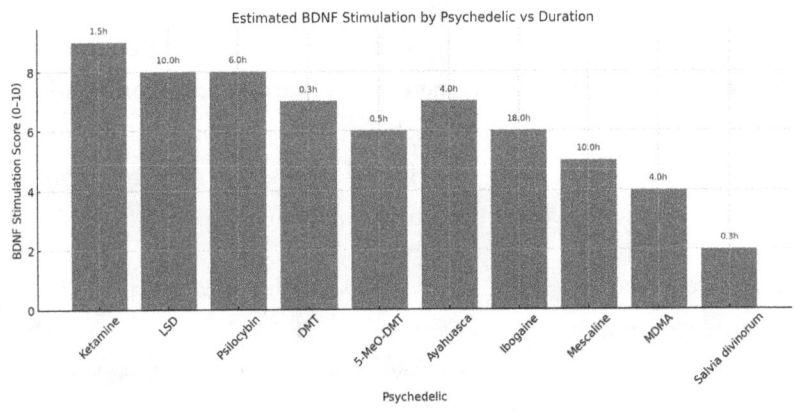

3. The chart above is an estimate of various psychedelics' impact on BDNF stimulation, along with typical duration based on existing studies. Ketamine is noted to provide the most robust short-term stimulation. Additional research is needed to confirm the most potent stimulators and safe combinations that could be used for even more robust boosting.

So what are the Brain-Boosting impacts of BDNF?

BDNF Effect	Mechanisms of Action
1. Promotes Synaptic Growth & Strengthening	- Increases the **formation of new synapses** (synaptogenesis). - Strengthens **existing connections** between neurons.
2. Supports Neurogenesis (New Neuron Growth)	- Stimulates the **birth of new neurons** in the hippocampus (important for memory). - Essential for **replacing damaged or lost neurons**.
3. Enhances Long-Term Potentiation (LTP)	- Strengthens **neuronal communication** by reinforcing synaptic efficiency. - Essential for **long-term memory formation and learning**.
4. Increases Dendritic Spine Density	- More dendritic spines = **greater neural connectivity** (i.e., more hands reaching out to each other). - Helps neurons form **stronger, more complex networks**.
5. Protects Against Neurodegeneration	- Reduces **cell death & oxidative stress**. - Low levels of BDNF are linked to **Alzheimer's, depression, and cognitive decline**.

In summary, BDNF benefits the brain by enhancing synaptic growth, neurogenesis, long-term potentiation, and dendritic spine density while protecting against neurodegeneration.

2. Increased Neuroplasticity

One of the most profound benefits of psychedelics is neuroplasticity. As mentioned above, BDNF helps with this. Many of you have likely read Michael Pollan's ground-breaking book, "How to Change Your Mind". In his book, he discusses our improved ability to be more creative and adaptive following a mushroom journey, saying, "Psychedelics open a window of mental flexibility in which people can let go of the mental models we use to organize reality."[12]

What exactly is neuroplasticity, and how do various psychedelics enhance it?

Neuroplasticity is the brain's ability to adapt, reorganize, and form new neural connections throughout life. This process allows the brain to learn, recover from injury, and adapt to new experiences. It can also help one recover from a traumatic experience, hence its application in PTSD.

A helpful analogy is a bonsai tree. The art and science of bonsai tree cultivation has been ongoing for 1000 years and originally began in China. Psychedelics can act like a Bonsai tree master, pruning old branches and promoting the growth of new ones. Tree nutrition, lighting, and showing love to the tree can also impact its longevity and new growth.

Meditation, which originated in India approximately 5,000 years ago and spread east to China, Japan, and other Asian countries, also offers opportunities for enhancing neuroplasticity and should be paired with many of the brain health-promoting activities mentioned in this book.

What are the various types of Neuroplasticity, and how do they impact our brain?

Synaptic Plasticity (Short-Term Changes)

Involves strengthening or weakening of synapses (connections between neurons). Here are some ways we can enhance synaptic plasticity beyond psychedelic therapy:

- **Dual N-Back Training:** Improves working memory by increasing dopamine release and synaptic efficiency. Stimulates both audio and visual sequences. Try it by visiting this page: https://brainscale.net/app/dual-n-back/training.

- **Neurofeedback:** May help indirectly with synaptic plasticity. More research is needed.

- **Mindfulness Meditation:** Temporarily enhances synaptic function in attention-related brain regions.

- **High-Intensity Interval Training (HIIT):** Boosts brain-derived neurotrophic factor (BDNF), which enhances synaptic activity.

- **Playing an Instrument:** Strengthens short-term synaptic connections by requiring quick adaptation to new patterns. Learn to play guitar! Or for me, I'm learning to play the Handpan drum!

- **Fast-paced problem-solving** (e.g., Chess, Sudoku): Encourages rapid synaptic adjustments in the prefrontal cortex.

Structural Plasticity (Long-Term Changes)

- The brain creates new neurons or rewires existing ones over time.

- Learning a second language can increase gray matter density (new neurons) in specific brain areas.

Functional Plasticity (Compensatory Changes)

- The brain reallocates functions to different areas, especially after injury.

- Stroke survivors may regain movement as other brain regions take over lost functions.

Metaplasticity

- Metaplasticity is often described as the "plasticity of plasticity." It's the brain's version of a tuning dial for the degree of plasticity. In simple terms, it's how your brain adjusts its capacity to change based on past experiences. Here's a gardening analogy: regular neuroplasticity is when you plant new seeds (new connections) or pull weeds (remove old ones). Metaplasticity is the condition of the soil - if it's too dry or too rich, it affects how well those seeds grow. If you've had a lot of stress or trauma (draught), the soil becomes less fertile, and planting gets harder. But if the environment is nurturing (like after sleep, exercise, or psychedelics), the soil becomes amenable to growth again.

How do psychedelics enhance plasticity? Psychedelics, such as psilocybin, LSD, DMT, and ketamine, improve **structural, functional plasticity and metaplasticity**, so enhancing **synaptic plasticity** with brain games, music, and meditation should always be part of your cognitive enhancement strategy too. Other forms of plasticity exist, but these are the main types.

How does Neuroplasticity happen at the cellular level?
Neuroplasticity happens via:

- **Neurogenesis** - The birth of new neurons, particularly in the hippocampus. The most important part of the brain for memory recall.

- **Synaptogenesis** - The process by which new synapses (connections between neurons) are formed in the brain. It is a fundamental mechanism of neuroplasticity.

  Another excellent analogy from nature:

  Our brain's synaptogenesis is similar to the mycelial network, which is an underground system of fungal threads (mycelium) acting like nature's internet, connecting plants, trees, and breaking down leaves, etc. This network allows fungi to exchange nutrients, signals, and even chemical messages with plants in a mutually beneficial relationship. Recent research suggests that mycelial electrical impulses resemble neural firing, with potential implications for memory-like or decision-making behaviors. Synaptogenesis, like the growth of hyphae, is guided by biochemical cues in the environment, such as BDNF in the brain or root exudates in soil. So cool! To learn more about the mycelial network, check out Paul Stamets' 2019 enlightening movie, "Fantastic Fungi."

- **Pruning** - The removal of unused or weak neural pathways.

- **"Use it or lose it" principle** - The more you engage in a skill, the stronger the neural pathways become; the less you use them, the weaker they get. For example, conversing in a foreign language so you maintain fluency.

So, how and why does "synaptic pruning" occur?

Overproduction of Synapses (Neurogenesis & Synaptogenesis)

- During early development and learning, the brain creates excess synapses to explore different neural pathways. For example, a child's brain has twice as many synapses as an adult brain at its peak because the excess synapses are pruned as they mature.

Tagging Weak Synapses for Removal
- Synapses that are rarely used or inefficient are marked for elimination. Microglia cells (your brain's immune cells) help detect underused synapses by recognizing low activity or weak electrical signals.

Microglial & Astrocytic Pruning (Neural Cleanup Crew)
- Microglia engulf and remove weak synapses through a process called phagocytosis (like "eating" neural debris). Imagine the old Pac-Man game.
- Astrocytes assist by regulating which synapses should be strengthened or removed.
- This process is similar to "decluttering" the brain, allowing strong connections to thrive.

Strengthening of Important Connections (Hebbian Plasticity)
- Synapses that are frequently activated get stronger (Hebb's Rule: "Neurons that fire together, wire together").
- Learning new skills, solving problems, and practicing habits reinforce essential neural circuits while the weak ones fade.

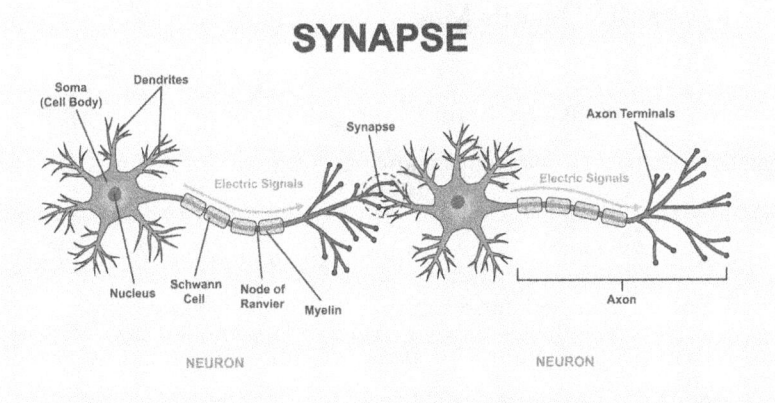

4. The Anatomy of a neuron and synaptic connection.

3. **Activation of 5-HT2A receptors supports brain health by**
    - Promoting the growth of new synapses and dendritic spines.

    - Supporting neuroplasticity and reducing neural inflammation

    - Repairing neural circuits disrupted by depression, anxiety, PTSD, and neurodegenerative diseases.

    - Helping to alleviate depression and anxiety.

    - Increasing openness to new experiences and improving recall and cognitive flexibility.

    - Helping to downregulate the default mode network (DMN), reducing ruminative and negative thought patterns.

    - Improving relationships, social bonding, and overall emotional intelligence.

4. Resets the Default Mode Network (DMN)

The DMN is a network of interconnected brain regions. It is often referred to as the brain's "autopilot" mode, responsible for daydreaming, self-awareness, and ruminative thinking that is active when you are not focused on the outside world. Psychedelics can reduce DMN activity, which may help people "get out of their heads" and feel more connected to the present moment or the world around them. So in short, reducing the DMN with psychedelics allows you to let go of both the things going on around you, as well as keeping you from going down a rabbit hole obsessing about things. It allows you to be present in the now. As emphasized in Ram Dass's book, "Be Here Now," and Eckhart Tolle's book, "The Power of Now." Our cell phone distractions, social media, and emails make it increasingly challenging to be in the present. Perhaps the reset of the DMN with psychedelics, particularly while in nature, will improve our nature-connectedness (as noted in studies) while also helping us simply be present and witness the beauty of a waterfall without a selfie involved. And of course, simply being more present with others.

Regions of the brain controlled by the DMN include:

Brain Region	Function in DMN
Medial Prefrontal Cortex (mPFC)	Self-referential thinking & decision-making
Posterior Cingulate Cortex (PCC)	Memory retrieval & internal reflection
Inferior Parietal Lobule	Spatial awareness & integrating sensory information
Hippocampus	Memory storage & consolidation
Lateral Temporal Cortex	Processing personal experiences & social understanding

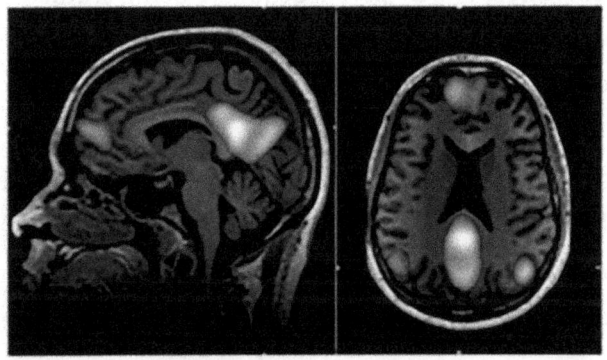

5. Default mode Network Regions (Wikipedia)

The **DMN is essential for self-awareness and memory, but excessive activity can lead to anxiety, overthinking, and depression.** Psychedelics, meditation, and immersive activities can help **reset the DMN**, leading to increased creativity, emotional breakthroughs, and personal transformation. It's easy for many of us to "go down the rabbit hole" and struggle with letting go of ruminating thoughts. As these patterned thoughts that can lead to spiraling depression are broken up, the frequency and severity of these episodes should be reduced.

How do Psychedelics Affect the Default Mode Network?

- Psychedelics like psilocybin, LSD, and DMT significantly reduce DMN activity.

- This allows for **more flexible thinking, enhanced creativity, and emotional breakthroughs.**

- The **DMN "shutdown" effect** is linked to ego dissolution, mystical experiences, and **neuroplasticity enhancement.**

- This effect is why psychedelics are being studied for **depression, PTSD, and addiction therapy**, where overactivity of the DMN plays a role.

How can I reduce DMN activity without Psychedelics?

- **Meditation & Mindfulness** - Shuts down self-referential thoughts and increases present-moment awareness.

- **Intense Exercise** - Reduces excessive self-focus and increases brain connectivity. (i.e. High Intensity Interval Training/HIIT)

- **Flow State Activities** - such as playing music or sports, fly fishing, or engaging in creative tasks suppress DMN activity.

- **Breathwork & Cold Exposure** - Techniques like **Holotropic Breathwork** lower DMN hyperactivity. Holotropic Breathwork is a therapeutic breathing practice developed by psychiatrist Dr. Stanislav Grof and his wife Christina Grof in the 1970s. It involves rhythmic, deep, and accelerated breathing combined with evocative music and bodywork, enabling individuals to access altered states of consciousness.

I like to tell my patients before a ketamine session that I'm going to "shake up your snowglobe". This is my analogy of how reducing the Default Mode Network (DMN) activity along with enhancing neuroplasticity, can help one shake loose intrusive, or stuck thoughts or fears, allowing them to settle into a healthier, more adaptive pattern. As mentioned earlier, Ketamine primarily achieves this by blocking NMDA receptors. Once the snow settles, it has repatterned itself to a degree, allowing them to let go of things that are, in a sense, trapped or held in by the DMN. Occasionally, during a Ketamine session, I'll witness patients letting go of a trauma, and may assist them with techniques such as breathing, sound-healing (with Tibetan bowls), and talk therapy to help them clear a trauma during the session. Follow-up integration sessions are recommended to everyone. Most of our patients have therapists who will delve deeper into integration following the sessions. Of course, trauma therapists are recommended for those who need them.

5. Enhances brain connectivity

Psychedelics allow the brain to enter a more flexible and interconnected state. This enhanced connectivity can lead to profound personal insights, emotional healing, and long-term changes in mental health. While I cannot find research to say that LSD increases "brain connectivity by 200%" or "brain wave QEEG activity by 300%," my opinion is that it does even more than that at higher doses. The fMRI in image 6 illustrates the enhanced brain connectivity from psychedelics. I have personally observed an increase in visual and acoustic acuity during psychedelic journeys, as most frequent users of psychedelics can attest. Whether it is appreciating the detail of a flower petal or hearing the tonal variations in a violin during a psilocybin journey, the difference is profound. I compare the visual acuity on psychedelics to an improvement one sees when you upgrade from a 1080P to a 4K TV.

Through the effects of neuroplasticity, the brain displays increased functional integration between brain regions and reduces constraints imposed by the default mode network (DMN). This leads to improved communication between normally segregated brain areas, including the Default Mode Network (DMN), the Salience Network (detects important stimuli), and the Central Executive Network (involved in conscious control and decision-making), which is thought to contribute to psychedelics' therapeutic and cognitive effects.

Researchers have found that psilocybin enhances communication between brain regions (see image 7) that typically don't interact, resulting in a more interconnected brain state.[13]

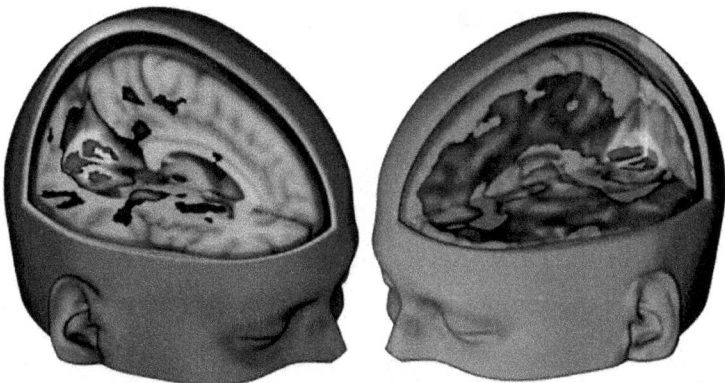

6. Researchers at the Imperial College of London discovered that large areas on fMRI associated with vision were more active and connected following the administration of LSD, as seen in the image on the right. This was also linked to hallucinations. Credit: Imperial College of London

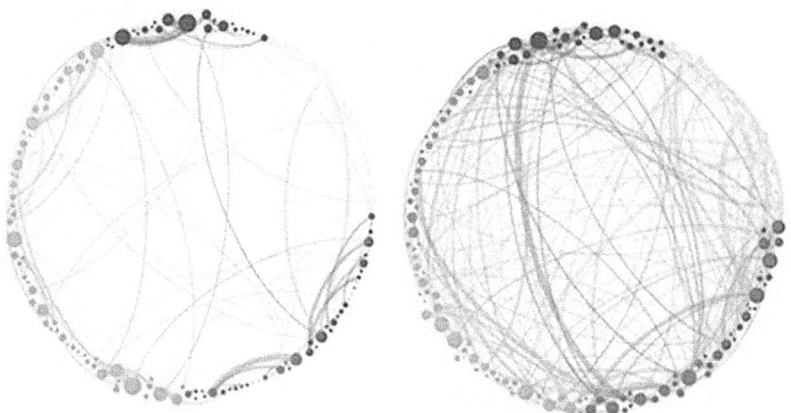

Image 7. Communication between functional brain networks in people given non-psychedelic compounds on the left, compared to those given psilocybin on the right. Credit: Petri et al., Proceedings of the Royal Society Interface.

6. Improves emotional memory processing (helping with trauma & PTSD)

Psychedelics enhance emotional processing by reducing activity in the amygdala, the brain's fear center, allowing individuals to face difficult emotions with less anxiety. They increase connectivity between emotional and cognitive brain regions, helping integrate past experiences with new insights. This often leads to emotional release, greater self-compassion, and a sense of resolution. By softening rigid thought patterns and ego boundaries, psychedelics foster openness, empathy, and improved emotional clarity.

7. Reduces Neural Inflammation

Psychedelics may reduce neural inflammation by interacting with serotonin 5-HT2A receptors, which are found not only on neurons but also on immune cells in the brain, like microglia. Activation of these receptors appears to shift microglia from a pro-inflammatory to an anti-inflammatory state, reducing the release of cytokines and other inflammatory markers. Specifically, they reduce levels of key pro-inflammatory cytokines, including interleukin-6 (IL-6), tumor necrosis factor-alpha (TNF-α), and interleukin-1β (IL-1β), as shown in preclinical studies and some human models. Studies in animals and cell cultures have shown that compounds like psilocybin, DMT, and LSD can decrease inflammation-related signaling pathways, potentially protecting against neurodegeneration and improving brain resilience. This anti-inflammatory effect may contribute to their therapeutic impact on depression, anxiety, and even neurodegenerative conditions.

8. Protects against memory decline (potential for Alzheimer's & dementia)

Psychedelics may protect against memory decline by enhancing neuroplasticity, reducing brain inflammation, and improving communication between key memory-related regions like the hippocampus and prefrontal cortex. They increase brain-derived neurotrophic factor (BDNF), promote synaptic growth, and reduce harmful cytokines such as IL-6 and TNF-α. By helping to reset rigid brain patterns and support emotional well-being, psychedelics create a more resilient and adaptable brain environment that supports healthy memory as we age.

The Critical Period

Outside of these eight, another benefit of psychedelics discovered recently is the opening of the Critical Period. Research on this benefit is just beginning, but the implications for brain function recovery, such as after a stroke, are encouraging.

After a psychedelic session, a **Critical Period** is opened. The critical period refers to a heightened window of neuroplasticity and psychological openness following a psychedelic experience, during which the brain is especially receptive to new insights, learning, and behavioral change. In general, the critical period is longer if the duration of the psychedelic effect is longer. Therefore, LSD and Ibogaine provide a much longer critical period than psilocybin. During this time, the mind and brain are more malleable, offering unique opportunities to rewire functional areas of the brain, reshaping thoughts, behaviors, and emotional patterns - more on this exciting new discovery in Chapter 5.

CHAPTER 2

Enhancing Cognition, Creativity, and Problem-solving with Psychedelics

As we age, it becomes increasingly challenging to think outside the box, and we may become more rigid in our opinions and thinking. Sometimes, we become more sensitive around specific topics. Dealing with prior authorizations for medications and imaging orders elicits a conditioned negative response from me.

For business professionals, participating in board meetings with younger leaders can become increasingly challenging. It's similar to going to the yoga studio and struggling to do a scorpion pose, especially when surrounded by those in their 20s. Well, honestly, I don't think I could have done that pose in my 20s. However, if we stretch our rigid muscles and encourage them with the help of a yoga instructor, we might impress ourselves and those around us.

Here are some real-world examples of enhanced creativity from psychedelics:

Watson and Crick DNA: James Watson and Francis Crick's discovery of **DNA's double-helix** structure in 1953 is thought to have been facilitated by Crick visualizing it on LSD.

Kary Mullis (Nobel Prize-winning chemist, inventor of PCR DNA amplification) openly credited LSD with helping him develop the **polymerase chain reaction (PCR)**, a breakthrough in genetic research. He said, *"Would I have invented PCR if I hadn't taken LSD? I doubt it."*

Steve Jobs shared his LSD experience, saying: "Taking LSD was a profound experience, one of the most important things in my life. LSD shows you that there's another side to the coin, and you can't remember it when it wears off, but you know it. It reinforced my sense of what was important - **creating great things instead of making money**, putting things back into the stream of history and of human consciousness as much as I could." He felt that Bill Gates would have been "more open-minded" if he had tried them. In general, he believed that his experiences with LSD likely played a role in his **unconventional thinking**, willingness to break norms, and intuitive design philosophy at Apple.[1]

Here are a few others you might recognize who have been positively impacted by the creative nature of LSD and other psychedelics:

Musicians:
- The Beatles (John Lennon, Paul McCartney, George Harrison)
    » Their music took a radical turn after their LSD experiences, leading to albums like *Revolver* and *Sgt. Pepper's Lonely Hearts Club Band*.
    » John Lennon: *"It opened my eyes. We only use one-tenth of our brain."*

- Jimi Hendrix, Janis Joplin, Pink Floyd, The Grateful Dead
  » Psychedelics were instrumental in shaping psychedelic rock and expanding musical creativity.

- Bob Dylan
  » Dylan was quoted in an interview saying, "*LSD is medicine*". The counterculture movement also influenced Dylan's music in the mid-'60s.

Writers & Philosophers

- Aldous Huxley (*Brave New World, The Doors of Perception*)
  » His book *The Doors of Perception* (1954) is a first-person account of taking mescaline, influencing the 1960s psychedelic movement.

- Terence McKenna (Ethnobotanist & Psychedelic Advocate)
  » Promoted psilocybin and DMT as tools for expanding human consciousness (Stoned Ape Theory).

- Hunter S. Thompson (*Fear and Loathing in Las Vegas*)
  » Psychedelic experiences heavily influenced his unique style of gonzo journalism.

Tech Visionaries

- Douglas Engelbart (Inventor of the computer mouse)
  » Participated in government-funded LSD experiments in the 1960s, which influenced his vision of human-computer interaction.

- Kevin Herbert (Cisco Engineer)
  » Described microdosing LSD as helping him solve complex engineering problems.

What has it done for me? Well, I haven't solved world peace, climate change, or discovered the meaning of life yet, but it has inspired me to write books and create innovative programs in my medical practice. Most importantly, it has provided a sense of dharma (universal and personal life duty) focusing on improving the health and wellness of others. It's allowed me to more intuitively assess a patient's health physically and emotionally as I can tune and focus on them rather than my brain being overburdened with allopathic medical thoughts. Medical conditions often stem from a deeper mind-body disconnect or unresolved emotional issues. I feel that having decades of psychedelic experience has heightened my sense of medical intuition.

How is it that creativity and problem-solving are enhanced with psychedelics and other mindfulness-based strategies?

It's a combination of several things already discussed. First, neuroplasticity and brain connectivity are enhanced. This happens through the stimulation of brain-derived neurotrophic factor (BDNF). There is also improved synaptogenesis (formation of new connections with neurons). A recent study at Johns Hopkins and the Imperial College of London found that psilocybin promotes new neural connections, helping individuals "break out" of rigid thought patterns.[2]

Also, as psychedelics take the Default Mode Network offline, it promotes a more fluid, creative mind with divergent thinking.

Divergent thinking enables us to think outside the box, with an enhanced ability to generate multiple ideas from a single prompt. For instance, what are the threats to the world if AI becomes sentient and lacks guardrails to prevent it from going rogue? I'm hopeful that more divergent human thinking will give us a deeper understanding of future AI threats.

See image 6, which demonstrates the vast increases in activity of the fMRI human brain before and after LSD, and electrical activity in the brain before and after psilocybin. The interconnectivity and brain wave activity (image 7) is multiple times what is found in a non-psychedelic state. It's this cross-brain communication that helps generate new unconventional associations and perspectives on life, as well as new insights into problem-solving and creative ideas. For me, LSD, mushrooms, Ayahuasca, and San Pedro have profoundly impacted my perception of patterns in nature, spirituality, relationships, global conflict, and so much more.

From the perspective of nature, I've found myself appreciating everything with greater depth and marveling at the beauty of its creation and evolution. Whether looking at the fractal geometry of brain coral on a dive, or recognizing the Fibonacci sequence/Golden Ratio in ammonites and the spiraling of a dissected pine cone, the heightened brain activity sparked by psilocybin and other psychedelics, for me, illuminates the sacred geometry woven throughout nature.

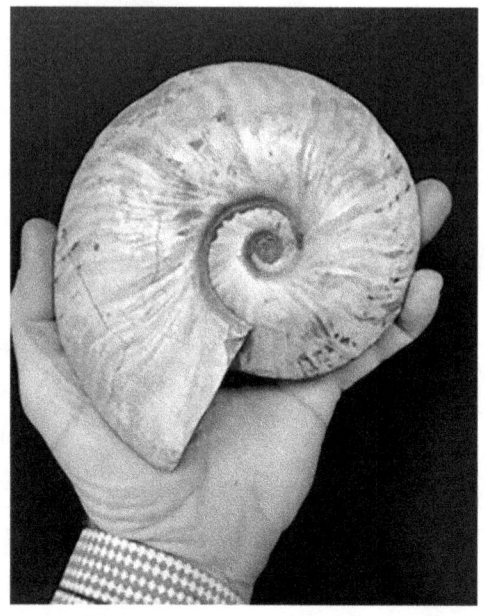
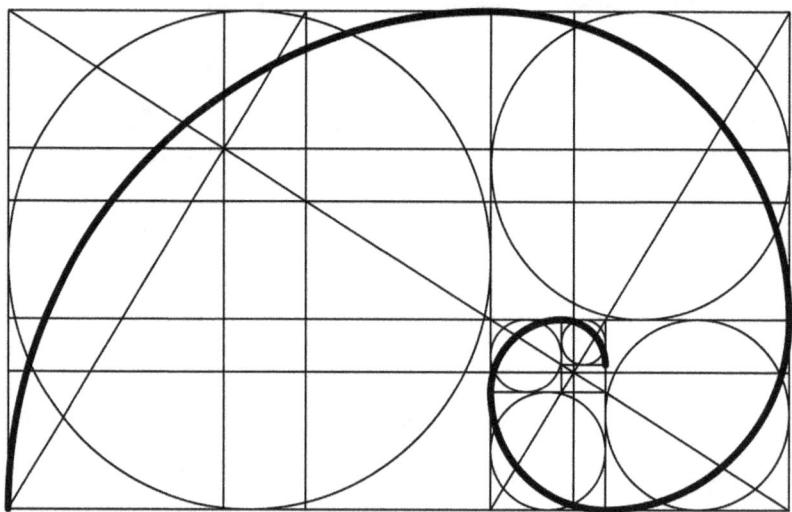

8. Ammonites and many other plants and animals contain the Fibonacci sequence, and Golden Ratio.

Sensory perceptions of taste, smell, touch, sound, and vision are markedly improved with psychedelics. The scent of juniper, the sounds of a mountain bluebird, and sensations of my hands dipping in a mountain stream are amplified as I hike the trails near my home in Durango. Psychedelics also promote convergent thinking. It's the ability to connect different ideas into a single practical solution or vision. Improved pattern recognition, lateral thinking, and insight problem solving (aha moment) help us crystallize a thought or solution. In a 1966 experiment by James Fadiman, he noted that psychedelics helped engineers and architects solve complex technical problems, leading to greater real-world innovation.[3]

In the fall of 2024, I went to Alex and Allyson Grey's home to see their new Entheon museum and attend a festive Halloween party for a long weekend. Alex and Allyson are the most prolific and well-known visionary artists in the world, finding much of their inspiration from LSD and other types of psychedelic journeys. I highly encourage everyone to see their art in the Entheon or at least online. While there, I met Martin Bridge, another amazing visionary artist who did the cover of this beautiful book. Their works, and those of many other artists in the genre, demonstrate the power of psychedelics in enhancing creativity, their understanding of nature, and the cosmos around us. Interdimensional realms are also revealed in ways that make us contemplate our origins, existence, and subtle energy fields around us.

In summary, psychedelics have helped visionary artists capture the world around us with a more intimate and spiritual perspective. These deep, creative insights would be unlikely to land on canvas without opening the "Doors of Perception" as per Aldous Huxley. I also believe that psychedelics can help us become better stewards of our planet's environmental health by promoting understanding and conflict resolution. The plant medicine teachers (psilocybin, Ayahuasca, San Pedro, Peyote, Ibogaine, etc) give us an opportunity for a greatly expanded vision, improved divergent and convergent problem solving, improved openness to potential solutions, and dissolution of barriers between humans, resulting in an enhanced collective consciousness as we come together, rather than seeing ourselves more divided. Divided we fail. Together, with the help of psychedelics, empathy, and altruism, we have the potential to thrive.

CHAPTER 3

Psychedelics for Mood Support, Anxiety, and PTSD

On a typical day at my medical practice, I manage, on average, three patients with anxiety and/or depression. Most are chronically struggling with this, but roughly 20% are newly diagnosed. Some may have more complex DSM-5 diagnoses, and oftentimes are being co-managed by psychiatrists and therapists in a team approach. The DSM-5 (Diagnostic and Statistical Manual of Mental Disorders, 5th Edition) is the standard classification system used by mental health professionals in the United States to diagnose psychiatric disorders. It is published by the American Psychiatric Association (APA) and provides criteria for diagnosing mental health conditions based on observable symptoms and behaviors.

Along with the ICD-10 (medical diagnostic codes), this cumbersome, time-consuming, unethical process of trying to get drugs and services approved by insurance using various codes is driving doctors nuts and pushing them towards early retirement. Many mental health disorders and medical disorders do not need to be subfractionated by seven alphanumeric categories. Insurance companies have weaponized the approval process by exploiting the complexity of ICD-10 coding to deny/game coverage, as providers painstakingly struggle and waste time filling out online forms with the exact codes to get something approved. If it's not approved, the doc has wasted at least 15 minutes of their time, and will be unlikely to write the prescription again. Insurance companies are increasing their profits by denying coverage for expensive medications, and sometimes denying even reasonably priced generic medications. Meanwhile, the patient often blames the provider rather than the insurance company, as they may not understand why their medication was denied.

As mentioned earlier, I have been unimpressed with the efficacy of antidepressants such as SSRIs and SNRIs. Common examples of prescribed medications in this class include Prozac, Paxil, Zoloft, and Wellbutrin. The effectiveness of these medications has been noted to be no better than a placebo, except in severe depression. Referral of my patients for psychotherapy has also been marginally successful. Most concerning has been the rise in suicidality amongst teens and adults. While I have lost less than six to suicide over my career, I always ask myself what I could have done better to prevent them. In all the cases, there were no red flags, no calls of desperation, just the unfortunate call from a loved one that they had taken their life. Some new patients with a diagnosis of severe depression would share that they still felt depressed on the four meds their psychiatrist prescribed, but didn't care about feeling that way. They were emotionally blunted (dissociated) to their depression and would walk into my office with a flat affect, seemingly disconnected from themselves and the world around them. Myself and many others feel that those who are blunted can be at risk for suicide. Hence, the black box warning on these psychotropics and the patient handout saying,

"May increase suicidality". One must question whether we are often doing more harm than good with these meds, especially when polypharmacy (multiple psych meds) is being deployed. When I see this, I carefully work with psychiatry to help them reduce doses, or the number of meds, and when feasible, legal, and safe with consent of all involved, I will often recommend microdosing of psilocybin, which I have found more effectively treats depression and anxiety and does not cause blunting. I am not totally against these medications, and do feel that SSRIs and SNRIs are very helpful for some when used conservatively, and monitored closely for improvement in mood, and anxiety reduction. Reflexively prescribing them to move on to the next patient, or adding more rather than trying another class, is potentially dangerous. I have unfortunately witnessed many patients coming to me with severe blunting and side effects when their prescribing doctor was unwilling to taper down, switch, or consider other options such as psychedelic medicine.

As of February 2025, the most recent comprehensive data on suicide rates in the United States is from 2022. In that year, **49,476 individuals died by suicide**, equating to an age-adjusted rate of 14.2 per 100,000 people.[1] This rate reflects a slight increase from 14.0 per 100,000 in 2021.[2]

This has unfortunately been the case of so many Veterans who take their lives from PTSD evolving to depression and suicidality. Roughly 50% of those suffering from PTSD develop depression.

According to the U.S. Department of Veterans Affairs' 2024 National Veteran Suicide Prevention Annual Report, an average of 17.6 veterans died by suicide each day in 2022. This figure has remained relatively stable since 2001, when the average was 16.5 per day. Notably, the highest recorded average was 18.4 daily veteran suicides in 2018[3]. In 2024, the rate of Veteran suicides was 18 per day and accounted for 20% of all suicides in the United States[4].

Unfortunately, we missed a huge opportunity to reduce these numbers with the FDA recently shooting down breakthrough MDMA therapy. More on this later.

A study conducted more than 20 years ago analyzed the postmortem brains of those who had committed suicide. What researchers found was that every subject in the suicide group had significantly lower levels of BDNF than controls.[5] Could low levels of BDNF be a more significant cause of depression and suicidality outside of the traditional serotonin model?

In my clinical experience, anxiety disorders generally respond more favorably to SSRIs, demonstrating noticeably greater efficacy compared to their more variable and often modest impact on depression. When needed, the sparing use of benzodiazepines like Valium or Xanax can be used, but with caution to avoid addiction and side effects.

According to the National Institute of Mental Health (NIMH), in 2021, approximately 21.0 million U.S. adults experienced at least one major depressive episode, representing 8.3% of all adults. The prevalence was notably higher among adult females (10.3%) compared to males (6.2%), and highest among individuals aged 18-25 (18.6%).[6]

A 2023 Gallup poll reported that 29.0% of U.S. adults have been diagnosed with depression at some point in their lives, a rise of nearly 10 percentage points since 2015. Currently, 17.8% of Americans report having or being treated for depression. The rates are higher among women, with 36.7% reporting a lifetime diagnosis, compared to 20.4% of men.

What's the point of sharing this data? If one-third have suffered or are suffering from depression, and almost 50,000 are committing suicide annually, then something isn't working. Our mental health care system, our safety nets, and pharmaceuticals don't seem to be doing enough.

Stressors/Situations that could tip suicidality into epidemic proportions in what some call "deaths of despair" could arise from:

- Increasing wealth disparity - an ever-wider chasm between working-class earnings and the soaring incomes of the economic elite.

- Ongoing inflation with no end in sight, especially with rising tariffs and the cost of goods being passed on to the consumer.

- Jobs lost to AI, or unethical downsizing by the government or corporate America.

- A lack of access to mental health services due to cuts in Medicare, Medicaid, and ongoing lack of coverage from insurance plans for these critical services.

- The uninsured or underinsured find little to no access to mental health care.

- Minimal access due to the legality and cost of healing psychedelic plant medicine and modern psychedelic molecules that are showing more hope than most modern pharmaceuticals.

- The stigma of seeking mental health treatment and untreated spiraling depression.

- Climate change and the recognition by youth that the future of planet Earth is grim at this point.

- Soaring educational costs - why bother getting a college degree and accruing massive debt if the planet is supposedly going to implode in 10 years? Even with a graduate degree, many are struggling to find a job, buy a house, pay off loans, or even afford food for themselves and their family members.

These are real concerns that are often not appreciated by the wealthy, especially those in the billionaire class, who are soon competing to achieve trillionaire status for egoic gratification while building rockets. My list above is a short one, but it could be pages long.

According to Visual Capitalist, "In 1989, the top 1% held **22.8%** of total U.S. net worth. As of 2024, this share has surged to **30.8%**. Although this figure has hovered close to 30% over the last decade, the overall rise underscores the growing concentration of wealth at the very top."[8]

In contrast, the bottom 50% of households collectively own about 2.5% of the total wealth.[9]

In summary, depression and anxiety are relieved by psychedelics as they promote neuroplasticity, reducing overactivity in the default mode network, and enhancing emotional processing. They can help reset rigid thought patterns, surface repressed emotions, and create profound shifts in perspective, often accompanied by feelings of connection, meaning, and inner peace. Biochemically, they affect serotonin and glutamate systems, with compounds like ketamine providing rapid relief. When combined with guided therapy, these effects can lead to lasting improvements in mood and mental health. Rather than blocking serotonin reuptake as with SSRI's, psychedelics do much more through the effects mentioned. I'm hopeful that psychedelics can help us reframe and cope with the ongoing stressors in our world today, reducing suicides and improving overall happiness.

The opportunity of psychedelics to effectively treat PTSD

In the fall of 2024, I attended a MAPS course online and at the beautiful Usona Institute (near Madison, WI) to become familiar with the future goal of becoming certified and approved to offer MDMA for the effective treatment of PTSD. Recent Phase 3 clinical trials conducted by Lykos showed the treatment had a 71% efficacy rating for PTSD.[10,11,12]

Unfortunately, despite completing the long course and learning how to perform MDMA therapy safely, it was shot down by the FDA several months later. While I'm hopeful to see it become approved, it will likely take at least a few more years. In my opinion, this delay in approval will lead to many more suicides of veterans and others who could have been saved by this breakthrough, effective therapy rather than the marginally effective current strategies. Sometimes, harm is caused by too much scrutiny by the FDA in our country, resulting in the loss of access to a safe and effective treatment. For example, Asia is rapidly and safely accelerating stem cell therapies, and I'm hopeful we can keep up with them given our ongoing restrictions.

Credit goes to Rick Doblin, MAPS (Multidisciplinary Association for Psychedelic Studies), and Lykos for their ongoing research and public education to help make this available eventually.

As mentioned earlier, MDMA (3,4-Methylenedioxymethamphet-amine) is often classified as an empathogen-entactogen rather than a traditional psychedelic, but it shares some characteristics with psychedelics.

MDMA primarily enhances **empathy, emotional openness, and social connection**, distinguishing it from classical psychedelics like LSD, psilocybin, and DMT, which mainly alter perception and cognition. It is often combined with low doses of LSD, psilocybin, and 2-CB to offer even greater depths of healing.

MDMA is a remarkable and profound molecule that increases serotonin, dopamine, and norepinephrine, resulting in euphoria, emotional warmth (heart-opening), and a reduction in fear. Like all of these molecules, it has to be experienced and can't be described. In my opinion, this molecule shines among the top five for its healing potential, but depending on the condition being treated, it can be number one.

I have witnessed dozens of friends and patients who have shared their stories of healing traumas, relationship issues, or simply letting go of unwanted energies with this molecule. MDMA can help reduce PTSD symptoms by promoting emotional processing and reducing fear.

MDMA was first synthesized in 1912 by Anton Köllisch, a German chemist working for the pharmaceutical company Merck. However, at the time, Merck was not interested in MDMA for its psychoactive properties.

Here is a brief timeline of the history of MDMA:

- **1912 - Anton Köllisch** synthesizes MDMA at Merck, but it is not tested for its psychoactive effects.
- **1927 & 1950s** - Merck scientists revisit MDMA, but it remains largely overlooked.
- **1960s - Alexander Shulgin**, a renowned American chemist, re-synthesizes MDMA and **tests its psychoactive effects on himself.** He notes its ability to enhance emotional openness and empathy.
- **1970s** - Shulgin introduces MDMA to psychotherapists, who begin using it in therapy to help patients process trauma.
- **1980s** - MDMA gains popularity as a recreational drug (Ecstasy) in party and rave culture.
- **1985** - The U.S. DEA classifies MDMA as a Schedule I drug, banning its medical use despite pushback from therapists.
- **2000s-2023** - Renewed interest in MDMA thanks to Rick Doblin, leading to its classification as a **break-**

- **through therapy for PTSD**, via successful clinical trials by MAPS and Lykos.

- **2024** - FDA rejects approval of MDMA for PTSD treatment by Lykos Pharmaceutical for controversial "safety and efficacy reasons". Many in the research and psychedelic community have voiced concerns about bias on the FDA panel and the potential influence of pharmaceutical companies who may have lobbied to protect assets of future sales of existing drugs (SSRIs) used for PTSD, seeing the obvious financial losses of an effective PTSD treatment with MDMA.

Given the recent radical changes coming to the FDA and other health care agencies, perhaps there is hope that another operation "Warp Speed" will occur for this potent healing molecule.

In the meantime, many will continue to seek MDMA therapy in the underground in desperation to alleviate their PTSD. While most underground facilitators and therapists using MDMA are well-trained and competent, there will be some outliers who pose risks to individuals. Careful screening, references, and recognition of the legal risks are critical for those seeking underground help before we get FDA approval. (Please note, I am not advocating for underground MDMA therapy.) Additionally, MDMA must always be checked for purity and for the purposeful or inadvertent contamination with fentanyl.

Once the FDA approves it, the risk of adverse events will decline as pharmaceutical-grade MDMA is available to qualified practitioners. For this reason, I'm hopeful that our country will expedite approval soon.

How do psychedelics promote emotional resilience?

Psychedelics, such as psilocybin, LSD, and MDMA, support **emotional resilience** and **mindfulness** by influencing brain function, neuroplasticity, and emotional processing. Here's how:

1. **Enhancing Emotional Resilience**

Emotional resilience refers to one's ability to adapt to stress, trauma, or adversity. It gives us a great ability to "bounce back" after going through trauma. Psychedelics can help with resilience via:

- **Neuroplasticity & Brain Connectivity**
    » As psychedelics promote neurogenesis and increase synaptic connections, particularly in areas like the prefrontal cortex and hippocampus, the brain can "rewire" itself, resulting in healthier responses to emotional stress.
    » Studies show that psilocybin enhances connectivity between different brain regions, which can break down rigid thought patterns and facilitate new, more adaptive ways of thinking.[13]

- **Processing Trauma & Fear Reduction**
    » **MDMA** and psilocybin help reduce the fear response by dampening activity in the **amygdala**, the brain's fear-processing center. The fight-or-flight response is less likely to be triggered unnecessarily.
    » This effect allows individuals to confront and process traumatic memories with reduced emotional distress, which is why MDMA is used and is often effective in **PTSD therapy**.

- **Increased Psychological Flexibility**
  - » Psychedelics encourage **cognitive flexibility,** helping people shift from negative or rigid thought patterns to more open, adaptive ones.
  - » This flexibility enhances the ability to **bounce back from challenges** and regulate emotions more effectively.

2. Supporting Mindfulness & Presence

Mindfulness is the ability to stay present and aware without excessive judgment or emotional reactivity. Psychedelics promote this in several ways:

- **Dissolving the Ego (Ego Dissolution)**
  - » Many psychedelics cause a **temporary weakening of the ego**, reducing the sense of separation between self and the world.
  - » This can enhance feelings of **interconnectedness, acceptance, "oneness," and a deep sense of presence.**
- **Increasing Awareness & Introspection**
  - » Psychedelics heighten awareness of thoughts, emotions, and bodily sensations, much like meditation.
  - » This increased self-awareness makes it easier to **recognize negative patterns and release unhelpful attachments.** This also helps to acknowledge how holding on to a resentment can cause harm, and then allows one to let it go. When I witness someone sharing the need to release a trauma or negative energy, such as a resentment, I often guide them

in breathwork to help release it, or may even help them clear it with energy work. This can be a rough process where crying and screaming may occur, but shifting them to breathwork and helping them move the energy more fluidly is my aim.

- **Encouraging Acceptance & Gratitude**

  » Many users report a greater sense of **acceptance and gratitude** after a psychedelic experience. MDMA in particular, promotes profound feelings of gratitude for being on this planet and also for the people around you. It enables individuals to more readily seek forgiveness, whether in couples therapy or simply while enjoying time together watching a sunset during an MDMA journey.

  » These effects can mirror and even enhance mindfulness practices by promoting **non-attachment to thoughts and emotions**. In a sense, you can see a painful thorn from your past, pull it more easily and effectively, let it go, and then feel lighter and happier following this process.

Synergies with Mindfulness-Based Practices

- Psychedelics and mindfulness meditation work well together, as both promote **present-moment awareness, emotional balance, and cognitive flexibility.**

- **Being in nature** while meditating or hiking on psychedelics can amplify the experience and provide for deeper healing as well. My personal favorite is to meditate by a mountain stream in solitude, or with a small group of like-minded individuals in nature. Just keep the mosquitoes at bay with some bug juice and clothing!

- Enjoying **music and sound healing** that is calming and resonates with psychedelic states.

- Individuals who engage in **meditation before or after psychedelic experiences** may experience **stronger and longer-lasting benefits.**

- Working with a therapist or trained psychedelic facilitator to help set intentions before and after a psychedelic ceremony/session is recommended for those who are working through traumas or other mental health issues.

Psychedelics facilitate emotional resilience by promoting neuroplasticity and flexible thinking, while enhancing mindfulness by increasing present-moment awareness and emotional acceptance. These effects have made psychedelics promising tools for mental health treatment, especially in conditions like depression, PTSD, and anxiety. They are also helpful in improving socialization among individuals and groups. It would be amazing to see a psychedelic retreat aimed at solving the Middle East and/or Ukrainian conflicts occur at Camp David. Dissolving their egos and enhancing their sense of empathy and connection would hopefully facilitate greater opportunities for problem-solving and peace. Sound crazy?! Well, look where we are today in the world - we are at a place where we need to stand more firmly for peace. In this modern world, we shouldn't be tolerating war crimes and genocide. We must come together boldly and not look the other way.

CHAPTER 4

Microdosing Psilocybin for Enhanced Cognition and Brain Health

There isn't a week that goes by when I don't have at least a few patients inquire about the benefits of microdosing. Some have heard about it from friends, social media, or from reading books like Michael Pollan's "How to Change Your Mind".[1]

The scientific evidence behind **microdosing psilocybin and LSD** is still evolving, with **mixed results** from clinical and observational studies. Anecdotal reports suggest benefits such as enhanced mood, creativity, and cognition, while more rigorous **placebo-controlled** trials often show more **modest or inconclusive** results.

I've noted benefits in mood, creativity, and cognition over the years while microdosing psilocybin. Typically, I do so for a few months on and a few months off, and have also interspersed it with occasional larger macrodose journeys, which may further amplify the benefits beyond simply microdosing. While I have not yet tried microdosing of LSD, I do feel that the longer duration of action would offer more substantial benefits.

Studies demonstrating the benefits of microdosing include:

Mood and Mental Health
- **Depression & Anxiety:** Some studies suggest microdosing could **reduce symptoms of depression and anxiety.**
  - » **Anderson et al. (2019):** A survey of microdosers found improved mood and reduced depression compared to non-microdosers.[2]
  - » **Prochazkova et al. (2018):** Found **enhanced creative thinking and problem-solving** abilities.[3]
  - » **Cameron et al. (2020):** In rats, microdosed LSD **increased stress resilience** and neuroplasticity markers.[4]

Cognitive Performance
- Some reports suggest **increased focus, problem-solving, and creativity.**
  - » **Hutten et al. (2020):** Microdosers reported **higher levels of attention and well-being,** but placebo-controlled studies are lacking.[5]

Neuroplasticity & Brain Health
- Microdosing may **promote neuroplasticity** by increasing **BDNF (Brain-Derived Neurotrophic Factor).**
  - » **Ly et al. (2018):** Showed that psychedelics **increase dendritic growth** and synaptic connections in neurons.[6]

Longevity

A groundbreaking 2025 study led by researchers at Emory University and Baylor College of Medicine found that psilocybin, through its active metabolite psilocin, may significantly slow biological aging by enhancing cellular resilience, reducing oxidative stress, preserving telomere length, and activating longevity-associated genes such as SIRT1. In human cell cultures, Psilocin extended cell lifespan by up to 57%, while aged mice treated monthly with psilocybin showed a 30% increase in survival and visible reductions in age-related decline. These findings suggest psilocybin could act as a systemic geroprotective agent, offering potential beyond its known mental health benefits, though human trials are still needed to confirm these effects.[7]

A great option to assess microdosing benefits to cognitive performance and mental health is the Microdose.me study app. I have recommended this to many patients who have made the decision to try microdosing for the potential benefits and would like to see some objective data. It's one of the most extensive global observational studies on microdosing psychedelics, conducted by Quantified Citizen in collaboration with researchers from the University of British Columbia, Maastricht University, and Macquarie University. The study collects self-reported data from thousands of participants who microdose psilocybin, LSD, and other psychedelics. The study primarily focuses on cognitive, emotional, and mental health outcomes.

Key Findings from the Microdose.me study have shown:

Improved Mental Health & Mood
- **Lower depression & anxiety scores** compared to non-microdosers.
- Older adults (>55 years) showed the most **significant reductions in depression.**

Cognitive Benefits
- **Improved psychomotor performance** in older adults.
- Potential **increases in creativity and problem-solving skills.**

Well-Being & Lifestyle Changes
- **Enhanced mindfulness and self-awareness.**
- Some participants reported **improved social interactions and emotional balance.**

Limitations & Caveats
- The study relies on **self-reported data**, which may introduce **bias.**
- There was **no placebo control**, meaning effects could be due to **expectation** rather than psychedelics themselves.
- Individual **dosages, frequency, and substances** vary, making it hard to generalize findings.

Microdosing Protocols

Below are a few of the common microdosing protocols. My preference is simply taking 100mg, four days on, three days off. I've found that many can be a bit overstimulated at 100mg-200mg, so 50mg can be a safer starting dose. Titrating up (gradually increasing the dose) can be done after a month of therapy if the desired results are not achieved. That being said, not all will feel the same at 100mg. Some mushroom strains have a much higher amount of psilocybin (thus also more downstream psilocin) than others, so starting low is best if you are not sure of the potency. Doing a larger three-gram or greater ceremonial drop once or twice monthly can be another option to consider if a microdosing regimen is not your style. Alternatively, doing a ceremonial drop-in session, then restarting microdosing one to two weeks later, is another reasonable approach. Everyone will have different needs in terms of dosing if they are treating depression and/or anxiety. Starting low and working up to find relief is best, but if you've given it three months at 200mg of psilocybin and you haven't seen results, you may consider increasing your dose. If that doesn't work, then perhaps you are a nonresponder. Nonresponders should talk to a psychedelic medicine professional to strategize options, which could include changing to a different strain or different psychedelic medicine, such as ketamine. Having a comprehensive functional medicine evaluation may be helpful as well. Perhaps you have a methylation issue or hypothyroidism that is blunting your response. For those taking rapamycin (Sirolimus) for antiaging purposes, consider taking it on the larger ceremonial day to prolong the "critical period" - more on rapamycin in Chapter 9.

Fadiman Protocol (by James Fadiman, PhD)
Dose: ~0.1–0.3 grams of dried psilocybin mushrooms, **taken every 4th day.**

Schedule
Day 1: Microdose

Day 2: Observation/Afterglow

Day 3: Rest (no dose)

Day 4: Microdose, Repeating the cycle

Stamets Stack (by Paul Stamets)
Dose: ~0.1–0.3g of psilocybin mushrooms

Stacked with: Lion's Mane (neurotrophic mushroom) and Niacin (Vitamin B3) - to enhance cerebral distribution via improved vasodilation and blood flow.

Schedule
Simply **4 days on**, 3 days off per week

Typically used for 4–6 weeks, followed by a rest period

Every Third Day Protocol
Dose: Same range (0.1–0.3g)

Schedule
Dose every 3rd day, allowing integration and avoiding tolerance buildup

I recommend following the Stamets Stack protocol 4 days a week, with optional Niacin, and taking it with Lion's Mane. Four weeks on, then two to four weeks off. What is Lion's Mane? Lion's Mane (Hericium Erinaceus) is a medicinal (non-hallucinogenic) mushroom known for its potential neuroprotective and nootropic (cognition enhancing) effects. It contains compounds like hericenones and erinacines that can stimulate nerve growth factor (NGF) production, which supports the growth, repair, and survival of neurons. Lion's Mane, like psilocybin, may enhance cognitive function, memory, and learning, and potentially protect against neurodegenerative diseases like Alzheimer's and Parkinson's.

Why is it important to take a microdosing break?
- Tolerance management - psilocybin tolerance builds fast; even microdoses can lose efficacy over time, so taking a break is essential, as shown in a cycle plan below.

- Neurochemical reset - Breaks allow serotonin receptors (especially 5-HT2A) to resensitize and become more responsive when restarted.

- Integration - Time off helps consolidate insights, emotional shifts, or cognitive changes.

- Safety - Long-term safety of continuous microdosing is not well established. Hopefully, with the opening of psilocybin centers in Colorado, we will have practice-based reporting of adverse long-term effects in the coming decade.

Here is an example of a Microdosing Cycle Plan

Week	Action
1–4	Microdosing (using a chosen protocol)
5–6	Break - no microdosing
7–10	Optional second cycle (or continue break)

While microdose.me is an ongoing observational study and doesn't provide conclusive evidence, it shows significant promise and should encourage additional, longer-term placebo-controlled trials. Again, funding for studies that don't have the potential to generate huge profits via a patented FDA-approved pharmaceutical drug is unlikely to happen. Unfortunately, the National Institutes of Health (NIH) budget for complementary medicine is being cut more as I write this. The NIH budget for **Fiscal Year (FY) 2024**, the NCCIH (National Center for Complementary and Integrative Health) received an appropriation of just **$170.3 million** and will likely be less moving forward.[8]

It will require more robust altruistic support from angel donors and philanthropists to support a trial of at least 1000 participants in a placebo-controlled, double-blinded study with standardized dosing of psilocybin to get confirmation of benefits, efficacy, and safety of microdosing. It would also be interesting to design more complex studies that look at cross-training the brain with psilocybin and LSD or others, by perhaps alternating the two on a monthly or weekly basis.

Additional adjunctive therapy, such as music therapy, guided meditation, AI-based neurofeedback, exercise, and other lifestyle changes, could be analyzed in subsequent trials or different arms of an extensive study.

What about psilocybin macrodosing vs microdose or a combination?

I enjoy a two to three gram deep dive once a month when time allows. These more profound experiences have allowed me to go inward, finding vision, clarity, and direction in my life. Oftentimes, I experience healing, which could be related to a trauma coming to the surface, allowing me to clear it with breath work, or having someone else volunteer to clear and balance my energy field. I've experienced messages from ancient ancestors, astral travel, and deep connections with nature in various journeys. Each experience is unique and varied, and I never know what to expect. Being in flow with the imagery, feelings, and incoming messages is critical for a good journey. If dark images or energies come in, I witness them and use my breath and sometimes my hands to energetically flow them into a black hole in the cosmos above. Re-centering with breath and grounding with my root chakra helps facilitate this as well. When the light energy comes in, I allow it to flow deep within my energy body. While this may sound crazy, once you have had enough deep dives with psychedelics, I trust you'll know what I'm referring to.

I've had a few patients with a terminal cancer diagnosis seek out a skilled end-of-life psilocybin facilitator to help them let go of their fear of death with great success. This is also helpful in reducing stress hormones (cortisol) and inflammation, likely leading to improved survival and an ability to be at peace with their circumstances. Larger doses of psilocybin, particularly in combination with low to medium doses of MDMA can also help treat PTSD, but studies are needed to confirm this observation. Below is a chart illustrating the differences between microdosing and macrodosing of psilocybin. Many are now microdosing LSD at 10mcg which can have a similar profile to psilocybin, but with a longer duration of roughly twelve hours instead of four.

Microdosing vs Macrodosing of Psilocybin

Feature	Microdosing	Macrodosing
Dose Size	0.1–0.3g	1–5g
Psychedelic Effect	Sub-perceptual	Strongly perceptual to mystical
Daily Function	Uninterrupted	Requires dedicated time & setting
Therapeutic Depth	Subtle, cumulative	Deep, transformative
Ideal Frequency	Four days/ week	Occasional (monthly or less)
Common Goal	Performance, mood, cognition	Healing, spiritual growth, reset

Legal and regulatory challenges of microdosing

While our society is tolerant of the ongoing staggering morbidity and mortality of alcohol, tobacco, opioid, and firearm-related deaths, we remain unwilling to fully legalize plant medicine that could help treat addiction, improve mood, cognition, and all the things we have discussed so far. Why the insanity? In my opinion, it has become a cultural norm to have and consume these mainstream harmful substances, or possess a firearm without a deeper appreciation or acknowledgement of the much higher likelihood of deaths related to each one.

Psilocybin, Ayahuasca, San Pedro, Peyote, MDMA, LSD, and other psychedelic-related molecule deaths over a decade are minimal, yet viewed as very harmful by those who haven't educated themselves on the real statistics. Most individuals, unfortunately, don't take even a few minutes to research the major harm of alcohol and tobacco compared to psilocybin. The chart below is worth a thousand words and should be appreciated by all, especially those who are against legalizing psilocybin in their states or nationwide. I'd love to see this plastered on billboards nationwide. Notice that the harm of alcohol even exceeds heroin and crack cocaine.

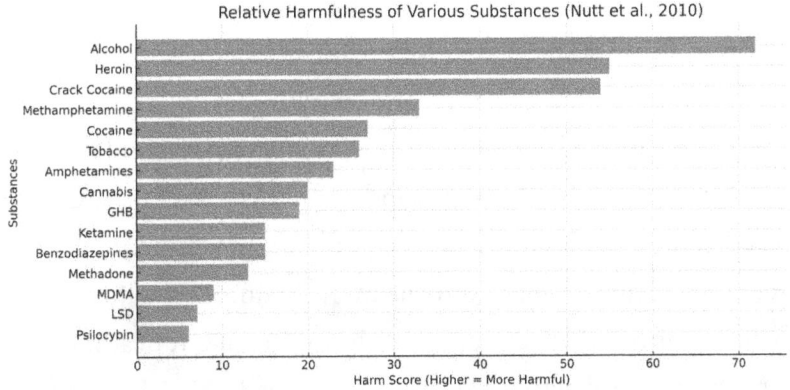

9. The chart above displays the relative harm of various substances based on the David Nutt et al. (2010) study. The harm scores consider both personal (e.g., addiction, health effects) and societal (e.g., crime, economic burden) impacts.

- **Alcohol** ranks as the most harmful overall due to its societal acceptance and widespread use.

- **Heroin and crack cocaine** are among the most harmful for individual users.

- **Tobacco and methamphetamine** also rank high due to health-related harms.

- <u>**Psychedelics like LSD and psilocybin**</u> are among the <u>**least harmful**</u> substances.

Brain Damage and Dementia related to Alcohol intake
According to a recent 2025 study in the Journal Neurology, researchers analyzed the brains of 1781 deceased patients (average age 75). They concluded that: Heavy drinkers who have eight or more alcoholic drinks per week have an increased risk of brain lesions called hyaline arteriolosclerosis, signs of brain injury that are associated with memory and thinking problems. Hyaline arteriolosclerosis is a condition that causes the small blood vessels to narrow, becoming thick and stiff. This makes it harder for blood to flow, which can damage the brain over time. It appears as lesions, areas of damaged tissue in the brain. After adjusting for factors that could affect brain health, such as age at death, smoking, and physical activity, heavy drinkers had 133% higher odds of having vascular brain lesions compared to those who never drank, former heavy drinkers had 89% higher odds, and moderate drinkers had 60%. Researchers also found heavy and former heavy drinkers had higher odds of developing tau tangles, a biomarker associated with Alzheimer's disease, with 41% and 31% higher odds, respectively.[9]

The "no-brainer" question to ask is: Why is psilocybin criminalized and unavailable in most states and countries, while alcohol is readily available everywhere and causing so much morbidity and mortality? Psilocybin should be available with minimal restrictions, especially since it and other psychedelics are showing significant promise toward the treatment of addiction disorders. In my opinion, it should be made available similarly to recreational and medical marijuana with a few extra guardrails. At most, make psilocybin Schedule 5, not a Schedule 1 drug under the Controlled Substances Act, and allow providers to screen for contraindications and prescribe safely, as I would for sending in a prescription for Prozac. According to Paul Stamets, most of us would have to consume **45 pounds** of psilocybin to be lethal. Compare that to drinking only one liter of vodka to take your life! Do you know anyone who has consumed 45 pounds of psilocybin to take their life or has had physical issues from the over-consumption of this non-addictive plant medicine? How many family members and friends do you know who have suffered mental, physical, and legal complications from alcohol? Do any of those kill others similar to drinking and driving? While I'm not for another prohibition of alcohol or outlawing guns, I do feel we need to see the big picture of relative harm from all of these substances. We need to exert greater control over the obvious legal things that are killing us, and make rational choices regarding improved access or decriminalization of low-risk plant medicines that may actually heal us. The same goes for Public health issues related to tobacco, narcotics, and guns, which would take another book to discuss.

Psilocybin was first **decriminalized** in Colorado in **2019** when Denver became the first progressive U.S. city to decriminalize personal possession and use through **Initiative 301**. I was happy to support Kevin Matthews, a U.S. Army veteran and activist who served as the campaign director of the Denver Psilocybin Initiative (DPI), a grassroots advocacy group. I advocated to as many patients and friends as I could to vote yes, along with many others, and it passed on the first round!

As of January 1, 2025, Colorado implemented significant changes regarding the legal status of psilocybin and certain other psychedelics. **Proposition 122**, which **decriminalized** psychedelic plants and fungi, including dimethyltryptamine (DMT), ibogaine, mescaline (excluding peyote), psilocybin, and psilocin, and set up a framework for legal, regulated use at licensed healing centers, became fully implemented in 2025 and allows for:

Personal Use and Cultivation:[10]
- **Legal Substances:** Individuals aged 21 and over may legally possess, cultivate, and use psilocybin, psilocin, DMT (dimethyltryptamine), ibogaine, and mescaline (excluding that derived from peyote).

- **Cultivation Limits:** Cultivation of psychedelic mushrooms is permitted within a private residence, limited to an area not exceeding 12 by 12 feet.

- **Sharing:** These substances can be shared among adults aged 21 and over; however, any form of sale remains illegal.

Regulated Therapeutic Use:
- Healing Centers: The state is in the process of establishing licensed "healing centers" where individuals can participate in supervised psilocybin sessions, expanding to other psychedelics in 2026. The licensing process for facilitators began on January 1, 2025, and as of July 2025, I know of two licensed centers that have opened in Denver, one of which is across the street from my office.[11]

Local Restrictions:
- **Municipal Authority:** While the state permits these activities, local governments have the authority to regulate or prohibit the establishment of healing centers within their jurisdictions. For example, Colorado Springs has implemented restrictions on such facilities, reflecting local policy decisions.[12]

Federal Law Considerations:
- **Federal Status:** Despite state-level legalization, psilocybin and similar psychedelics remain classified as Schedule I substances under federal law, indicating no accepted medical use and a high potential for abuse. This federal classification means that possession, cultivation, or use of these substances could still lead to federal legal consequences.[13]

Oregon enacted similar legislation in November 2020, becoming the first state to both decriminalize psilocybin and legalize it for supervised therapeutic use. This initiative, known as Measure 109, allows adults aged 21 and over to access psilocybin services at licensed facilities. The program officially began in 2023. Other states have various cities that are decriminalized, but not the whole state. These currently include: California, Michigan, Massachusetts, Washington, Minnesota, Maine, and Washington DC. Please check this Wikipedia page for updated status: https://en.wikipedia.org/wiki/Psilocybin_decriminalization_in_the_United_States

It's essential to stay informed about the legal status of plant medicines and psychedelics in your state, city, or country you are visiting. So please don't bring your psilocybin to Singapore unless you are willing to risk a long prison sentence or even the death penalty.

CHAPTER 5

The Potential of Psychedelics to Treat Neurodegenerative Diseases

In the preceding chapters, we've discussed the myriad of potential benefits from psychedelics' stimulation of various pathways that promote neuroregeneration and reduce inflammation. How might psychedelics help prevent or reverse Alzheimer's, and could they offer similar benefits for Parkinson's and other neurodegenerative conditions? So far, neuroscientists see promise, but ongoing long-term studies are needed to confirm these potential benefits. Funding, greater awareness, and acceptance of psychedelic medicine are needed to move this forward at a faster pace. We are likely looking at another decade of research to have these answers, so for many of us past the half-century mark, we have to make a proactive choice on whether the benefits outweigh the risks of deploying psychedelic therapies before large randomized controlled trials are completed. That is, if they are ever even funded and completed. Much of what I am sharing is to help individuals make that personal decision.

Early detection in any disease state is tantamount, as is identifying the early symptoms of Alzheimer's. This is becoming easier now, but it still takes a fair amount of proactive engagement from the individual or family members to begin an assessment. Many are afraid to take this path due to obvious fears of being labeled as potentially early Alzheimer's and the stigma and stress that may come with it. Identifying a red flag for early Alzheimer's can be seen as an opportunity to reverse or stave it off rather than giving in to potential cognitive decline. Again, the key is early identification and intervention for neurodegenerative conditions. Once someone has reached a more moderate stage, the opportunities to improve cognition are more limited. If you or your family members are concerned about potential cognitive impairment, there are many options available as I've listed below. Seeing your physician is best, but if you'd like to do some pre-visit testing on your own, there are online tests that can be done at home and then shared with your primary care and/or neurologist. These include:

Clinical & Cognitive Assessments are the first step:
- **MMSE (Mini-Mental State Examination)**

- **MoCA (Montreal Cognitive Assessment:)** more sensitive to early cognitive changes

- **Online home testing:** Since it can take several months to see a neurologist these days, I often advise my patients to consider a validated online test to pre-screen. Tests to screen for cognitive impairment and early signs of Alzheimer's include BrainTest®, a self-administered SLUMS-based tool with clinician review; CogniFit, offering a scientifically validated cognitive assessment and training; and the SAGE test from Ohio State, a printable exam used by doctors. Creyos provides in-depth, research-grade cognitive testing, while the Alzheimer's Association offers quick memory checks and education. These are then shared with the neurologist if they decide to go ahead with the referral.

- **Neuropsychological testing:** a detailed assessment of memory, attention, language, and executive function is often part of the formal evaluation.

Brain Imaging (along with Biomarkers is step 2)

- The most advanced imaging for Alzheimer's is the **amyloid PET scan**, which detects amyloid plaques in the brain, often years before symptoms become severe. Tau PET scans and FDG-PET offer additional insight into disease progression and brain metabolism. MRI is commonly used to assess brain atrophy and rule out other causes of dementia, making it a valuable first-line imaging tool in clinical practice.

Biomarker Testing (CSF and Blood) to determine risk of Alzheimer's.

Cerebrospinal Fluid (CSF) biomarkers that indicate an increased risk:

- Decreased levels of **Amyloid-beta 42 (Aβ42)**
- Increased levels of **Total tau (t-tau)**
- Increased levels of **Phosphorylated tau (p-tau)**

Blood-based biomarkers:

- **Plasma p-tau181 or p-tau217** – early indicators of tau pathology

- **Neurofilament light chain (NfL)** – a marker of neuronal injury

- **Plasma Aβ42/Aβ40 ratio** – correlates with brain amyloid levels.

- **Glial Fibrillary Acidic Protein (GFAP)** – an indicator of ongoing brain inflammation.

I offer the **PrecivityAD® test** in my office, which measures combined Aβ42/40 and p-tau217/np-tau217 (%p-tau217) ratios and ApoE genotype to estimate brain amyloid burden with high accuracy. It closely aligns well with PET scan results. Mayo Clinic and others offer it. It's pricey at roughly $1750, but they offer some aggressive discounts based on your income. This test is rarely covered by insurance.[1]

Whether you're at an increased risk of Alzheimer's or not, can psychedelics help prevent or reverse Alzheimer's?

Psilocybin, LSD, and DMT are being explored for their potential neuroprotective effects and ability to prevent or slow Alzheimer's disease. I am hopeful to see trials looking for the reversal of Alzheimer's in the future as well. At the very least, I feel that psychedelics can slow the progression.

Putting this all together, the mechanisms of neuroplasticity, regeneration, reduced inflammation, enhanced clearance of Amyloid and Tau Proteins, improved cerebral blood flow, improved mood (reduced anxiety and depression), stress reduction, and enhanced cognitive flexibility gives us a powerful opportunity to reverse or stabilize Alzheimer's.

Here are a few interesting ongoing studies:

1. Johns Hopkins University Study on Psilocybin for Depression in Early Alzheimer's Disease

Researchers at Johns Hopkins University are conducting a study to assess the efficacy of psilocybin-assisted therapy in treating depression among individuals with early-stage Alzheimer's disease or mild cognitive impairment (MCI). The study involves administering psilocybin in a controlled setting, accompanied by counseling sessions, to evaluate its impact on mood and cognitive function. Interested individuals can find more information or participate by contacting the research team at (410) 550-5466.[2]

2. Eleusis Ltd.'s Research on LSD Microdosing

Eleusis Ltd., a pharmaceutical company, is exploring the potential of microdosing lysergic acid diethylamide (LSD) as a treatment for Alzheimer's disease. Their research focuses on the anti-inflammatory properties of psychedelics, aiming to develop therapies that could mitigate neuroinflammation associated with Alzheimer's. The company is also investigating other psychedelic compounds for their therapeutic potential in neurodegenerative diseases.[3]

3. Akome Biotech's combined synthetic and plant medicine psychedelic compound in development

AKO-002 is a new compound in pre-clinical trials being developed by Akome Biotech for the treatment of Alzheimer's disease. It's a combination of a non-selective serotonin receptor agonist and the serotonergic psilocybin, as well as an undisclosed specific plant bioactive. Their data analysis and mapping have revealed evidence that psychedelics promote neuroplasticity and neurogenesis and act as agonists at serotonin receptors, including the 5HT2A receptors (5HT2A-R), that appear in high concentrations. These are in regions of the brain that are vulnerable to Alzheimer's, such as the hippocampus, which is critical for memory. Additionally, they have confirmed that psychedelics have been shown to have potent anti-inflammatory properties, and given their affinity for the 5HT2A-R, may represent a unique anti-inflammatory overwhelmingly targeted to brain tissue. Akome's plant bioactive appears to function synergistically with the psilocybin compound, exhibiting multiple mechanisms of action, including β-amyloid reduction and increased cerebral blood flow.[4]

Noted Biomarker Changes that may help reduce Alzheimer's Disease pathology

Benefit	Description/Implication
↑ Synaptic Protein Expression	Supports synaptic plasticity and communication between neurons
↑ Dendritic Spine Density & Branching	Enhances connectivity and complexity of neural networks
↓ Neuroinflammation	Reduces chronic brain inflammation that contributes to cognitive decline
↓ Amyloid and Tau Pathology (Preclinical Evidence)	Potentially prevents or reverses hallmark protein accumulations of Alzheimer's
Mood Enhancement	Improves emotional well-being, which may indirectly support cognitive function and resilience

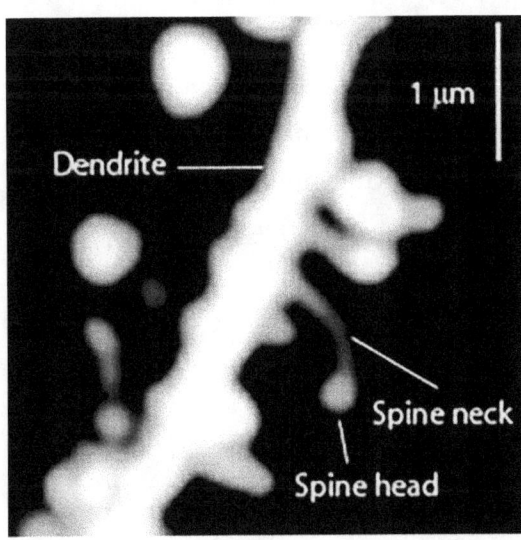

10. The number of dendritic spines (bumps on dendrite) can increase with psychedelic therapy as seen in this image. More spines=more neural connections. (Source: Wikipedia)

In summary, additional preclinical animal studies and AI modeling may provide a foundation for future clinical trials aiming to translate these findings into therapeutic interventions for Alzheimer's patients. I'm excited to see biotech companies combining ancient plant medicines with modern molecules in an alchemical way to potentially create more pronounced effects on brain regeneration, neuroplasticity, and inflammation reduction. Somehow, the Shipibo shamans of Peru magically discovered in their primal rainforest lab that combining the root of the ayahuasca plant with the chacruna shrub allowed DMT to stay active for a four-hour-long healing journey. The probability of finding the synergy of two distinct plants and creating this shamanic brew is one in a trillion based on AI calculations. Keep in mind that there are more than 40,000 plant species in the rainforest of South America. The cool, but bitter maroon colored plant extract is served sacredly in a shamanic circle, producing one of the most profound, psychoactive, and psychedelic experiences one could imagine. Modern progressive researchers who appreciate, respect, and understand the realms of ancient and contemporary shamanism have the most significant opportunities to discover and design new combinations that can maintain this wisdom and potentially take it to new realms. They must go beyond the conventional research models to do so, however.

Psychedelics for Parkinson's Disease

Parkinson's Disease (PD) is a progressive neurodegenerative disorder that affects movement. It occurs when dopamine-producing neurons in a part of the brain called the substantia nigra become damaged or die. Dopamine is a neurotransmitter essential for smooth, coordinated muscle movement. Loss of dopamine leads to the hallmark motor symptoms of Parkinson's, which can include tremors, slowed movement, muscle stiffness, and shuffled gait. Mental health symptoms can include depression, anxiety, and memory issues, to name a few. Trying to help patients with neurodegenerative conditions such as Parkinson's and Multiple Sclerosis has been challenging, with limited results, even with the assistance of the best neurologists and the latest medications available.

Psychedelics are being explored in the context of PD, primarily focusing on their potential to alleviate non-motor symptoms such as depression and anxiety, as well as their neuroprotective properties. Early in my career, I testified in support of stem cell therapies for PD while it was in the Health Care Committee at the Colorado State Capitol. Many were there opposing it, falsely assuming that aborted fetuses were going to be used as a source. Unfortunately, multiple barriers in our country have slowed research in this area, including limited funding, FDA headaches, ethical, religious, and political challenges, to name a few. Like other neurodegenerative diseases, it will take more public and private funding (i.e., Michael J. Fox Foundation) and expedited timelines to move it forward. Japan and Sweden are more likely to find a breakthrough via stem cell therapy than the US, in my opinion. However, in regards to the application of psilocybin, we are leading the way.

1. Psilocybin Research for Depression in Parkinson's Disease

Depression is a common non-motor symptom in PD, significantly impacting patients' quality of life. Researchers at the University of California, San Francisco (UCSF), are conducting a randomized controlled trial to assess the efficacy of psilocybin therapy in treating depression among individuals with PD. The study involves administering psilocybin in a controlled setting, accompanied by counseling sessions, to evaluate its impact on mood and cognitive function. This trial also examines the effects of psilocybin on neuroplasticity, which could have implications for both motor and non-motor symptoms of PD.[5]

2. Psilocybin's Anti-Inflammatory Potential

Silo Pharma, in collaboration with UCSF, conducted a clinical trial investigating the impact of low doses of psilocybin, assessing anti-inflammatory activity in people with PD. Reducing inflammation may reduce the progression of PD. Participants underwent preparation sessions, psilocybin dosing sessions, and integration sessions, with blood samples collected to assess the psychedelic's effect on inflammation.[6] In my office, we also use medical-grade curcumin, CBD, and glutathione to reduce neural inflammation. Perhaps a combination of psilocybin/curcumin/CBD/glutathione could be researched in future trials to determine the best combinations for optimal outcomes. Of note, if you are taking higher doses of curcumin, I recommend having your liver enzymes checked since it can cause liver inflammation in rare cases. GLP-1 peptides (i.e., Ozembic, Mounjaro) therapy for weight loss and diabetes therapy are also showing immense anti-inflammatory promise via reduction in proinflammatory cytokines. More on this later!

3. Psychedelics and Neuroprotection

As mentioned, preclinical studies suggest that psychedelics may promote neuroplasticity and synaptogenesis, indicating potential neuroprotective effects. These properties are relevant to neurodegenerative diseases like PD, where neuronal atrophy and synapse loss are prominent. While direct evidence in PD models is limited, the ability of psychedelics to stimulate neuronal growth and reduce inflammation warrants further investigation.[7]

Several clinical trials are underway to assess the safety and efficacy of psychedelics in treating PD symptoms. For instance, a Phase 1/2 clinical trial is investigating N,N-Dimethyltryptamine (DMT) as a potential treatment for Parkinson's disease. Additionally, Akome Biotech is developing a DMT-based formulation (AKO-004) targeting PD, which is currently in preclinical stages.[8] I'm hopeful to see additional trials exploring microdosing of ketamine therapy and LSD as well.

Supporting the anti-inflammatory pathways more comprehensively via psilocybin, glutathione, curcumin, and CBD, while also supporting mitochondrial function via methylene blue, NAD+ and Co-Q10 makes sense and deserves further investigation in my opinion. More on the complementary and synergistic molecules later!

Psychedelics for Multiple Sclerosis

Multiple sclerosis (MS) is a chronic, autoimmune disease that causes the immune system to attack the protective covering (myelin) of nerve fibers in the central nervous system (brain and spinal cord). This results in inflammation and damage to the nervous system that disrupts communication between the brain and the rest of the body.

Luckily, there's promising new research exploring the potential of psychedelics in treating MS. Similar to Parkinson's, it is focusing on their anti-inflammatory and immunomodulatory properties.

Significant anti-inflammatory effects were noted in preclinical studies looking at psychedelics via their serotonin 5-HT2A receptor agonist action. These substances may modulate immune responses without broadly suppressing the immune system, suggesting potential therapeutic applications for autoimmune and chronic inflammatory conditions like MS.[9] In doing so psilocybin reduces inflammation by downregulation of pro-inflammatory cytokines such as TNF-α, IL-6, and IL-1β, calming microglial overactivation, and improving stress response - all of which contribute to a system-wide anti-inflammatory effect.

In 2024, the European Union initiated a clinical trial to assess the effects of psilocybin in patients with progressive diseases, including MS. This study aims to evaluate whether **psilocybin can alleviate psychological distress** associated with incurable diseases. Approximately 100 patients are participating across sites in the Netherlands, Portugal, the Czech Republic, and Denmark.[10]

At the Johns Hopkins Center for Psychedelic and Consciousness Research, at the forefront of investigating psychedelics' therapeutic potential, studies have primarily focused on conditions like depression, anxiety, and addiction. The center's work contributes to a broader understanding of how psychedelics might be applied to various medical conditions, potentially including MS in the future.[11]

Recent studies have shown that psilocybin can cause significant changes in brain connectivity, resulting in the desynchronization of neural networks.[12] In my opinion, these changes may also underlie further therapeutic effects observed in mood disorders and could have implications for neuroinflammatory conditions like MS, more research is needed.

Ongoing Research and Future Directions
While current research is promising, it's still in the early stages. Further studies are necessary to fully understand the safety, efficacy, and mechanisms by which psychedelics might benefit individuals with MS. As research progresses, these substances could potentially be integrated into comprehensive treatment strategies for MS, pending rigorous clinical validation.

Imagine designing a trial that could include analyzing effects of multiple therapies, such as utilizing stem cell therapy for Parkinson's, reducing inflammation with psilocybin, while promoting mitochondrial function with NAD+ and methylene blue. There are so many powerful interventions to explore, but of course, the challenge is funding and more outside-the-box creativity for research design.

Psychedelics for Traumatic Brain Injury & Chronic Traumatic Encephalopathy

Emerging research indicates that psychedelics may offer therapeutic benefits for individuals with traumatic brain injury (TBI) and Chronic Traumatic Encephalopathy (CTE). They are being studied for their potential to promote neuroplasticity, reduce neuroinflammation, and improve cognitive and emotional functioning, similar to how they may help conditions such as PD, MS, Alzheimer's, and those of us without disease.

TBI is a disruption in normal brain function caused by a blow, jolt, or penetrating injury to the head. It can range from mild (like a concussion) to severe, potentially causing long-term disability or even death. Most of the TBIs I see in Colorado are sports-related due to biking accidents and skiing. Motor vehicle accidents are another prevalent cause even from whiplash alone without a blunt impact.

CTE is a progressive neurodegenerative disease associated with repeated head injuries, commonly observed in athletes (Boxers and Football players, especially) and military personnel. Currently, there is no definitive cure for CTE, and treatments primarily focus on managing symptoms.

Emerging research suggests that psychedelics, such as psilocybin and Ibogaine, may offer potential therapeutic benefits for individuals with traumatic brain injuries (TBIs), which share pathological similarities with CTE.[13]

As mentioned earlier, numerous psychedelics have been shown to promote neuroplasticity. This rewiring property is particularly relevant for conditions like TBI, where neural pathways are damaged. TBI and CTE likely benefit from the modulation of neuroinflammation, hippocampal neurogenesis, and neuroplasticity.[14]

There are individual cases suggesting potential benefits of psychedelics for brain injuries. For instance, former UFC fighter Ian McCall reported significant improvements in his TBI symptoms after undergoing psilocybin therapy. McCall's experience underscores the potential of psychedelics in addressing neuropsychiatric symptoms associated with repetitive head trauma.[15]

There are also **anecdotal reports** of potential benefits of Ibogaine for TBI. In a 2024 TBI study published in Nature, 30 combat veterans studied demonstrated that a single dose of Ibogaine improved symptoms of TBI, post-traumatic stress disorder (PTSD), and other related conditions.[16] Ibogaine is also showing promise in the treatment of addiction disorders, particularly for opioid and heroin addiction. Most are seeking Ibogaine therapy in Mexico, but there is also a center in Portugal. To be accessible and affordable to many, I am hopeful that Colorado will open a treatment center in 2026 or earlier.

Preclinical research with psilocybin in rodent models has demonstrated that psilocybin could restore brain function after mild, repetitive head injuries to female rats. The study found that psilocybin treatment reduced brain swelling and improved functional connectivity between brain regions further suggesting a potential therapeutic role for psychedelics in treating head trauma.[17]

While preclinical studies and anecdotal evidence are promising, rigorous clinical trials are necessary to establish the safety and efficacy of psychedelics for treating CTE specifically. Researchers are exploring various psychedelics for their neuroprotective and neuroregenerative properties, aiming to develop novel treatments for neurodegenerative diseases. For instance, the UC Davis Institute for Psychedelics and Neurotherapeutics, led by David E. Olson, is investigating the therapeutic potential of psychedelics in treating conditions like CTE.[18]

The potential of psychedelics as therapeutic agents for TBI and CTE is an emerging area of research as with other conditions. Preliminary findings indicate that ancient plant medicines like psilocybin and Ibogaine may promote neuroplasticity, reduce neuroinflammation, and improve cognitive function following brain injuries. However, comprehensive clinical studies are required to validate these effects and determine appropriate treatment protocols. My personal opinion is that some individuals may want to do a trial of microdosing psilocybin along with other conventional therapies under the guidance of their physician or a provider with psychedelic expertise to see if symptoms improve. Of course, they must be aware of the unknown potential risks while recognizing an opportunity to heal. Later in this book, I will also discuss the benefits of near-infrared light therapy that can be used in combination with psychedelics and methylene blue to help further regenerate the brain and aid in recovery.

The Benefits of Psychedelics in Stroke Recovery

Most of us have known a family member or friend who has suffered from a stroke. I've even had a friend who suffered one in his 30s, and luckily, I have only seen a few in my practice over the years. I make a strong effort to keep my patients' blood pressure under control, as well as limiting other cardiovascular risk factors through advanced screening.

Currently, it is estimated that more than 795,000 individuals experience a stroke each year. Of these, approximately 610,000 are first-time strokes, while about 185,000 occur in individuals who have previously had a stroke. Ischemic strokes, which result from blocked blood flow to the brain, account for roughly 87% of all stroke cases.[19]

Acute stroke, if treated early with intravenous thrombolysis using tissue plasminogen activator (tPA) and in some large vessel clots treated with mechanical thrombectomy, can allow some to recover with less long-term damage. The key is rapid identification of a stroke and treatment. **Every minute without treatment=millions of neurons die.** Only about 10–15% of stroke survivors recover completely with no lingering symptoms (either physical, cognitive, or emotional). The other 85-90% need ongoing therapy and often are entirely dependent on care from others for daily living. Improved prevention, early detection, and rapid treatment are critical, and we must explore more effective therapies for psychedelic stimulation and stem cell therapies to promote regeneration and rewiring post stroke.

Clinical Trials Investigating DMT for Stroke

Luckily, several clinical trials are underway to assess the safety and efficacy of DMT in stroke treatment. They include:

- **Algernon NeuroScience Phase 2 Study**: Algernon NeuroScience has finalized a clinical trial design for a 40-patient Phase 2 study investigating an intravenous sub-psychedelic dose of DMT in patients hospitalized after an acute ischemic stroke. This study aims to explore DMT's potential to promote neuroplasticity and aid in brain injury healing.[20]

- **Phase 1 Safety Study**: The same company has initiated a Phase 1 clinical study to evaluate the safety, tolerability, and pharmacokinetics of DMT when administered as an intravenous bolus followed by prolonged infusion. The first subject has been dosed in this study, marking a significant step towards understanding DMT's therapeutic potential in stroke recovery.[21]

Research Initiatives at Academic Institutions are also exploring the role of psychedelics in enhancing neuroplasticity in stroke patients:

- **Johns Hopkins University (JHU) PHATHOM-Stroke Project**: Researchers at JHU are investigating whether combining psychedelics with physical therapy in digitally enriched environments can restore motor function in stroke patients, even in cases where the stroke occurred months to years prior. This study aims to provide critical data on patients' willingness to use psychedelics and adopt digital therapies.[22]

- **Johns Hopkins Study on Critical Periods:** A study conducted at Johns Hopkins Medicine demonstrated that psychedelic drugs could reopen "critical periods" for social learning in mice. These periods are times when the brain is particularly receptive to learning new skills, suggesting potential applications in stroke rehabilitation.[23]

How do psychedelics help in stroke recovery?

Several mechanisms are thought to be involved and include:

- **Sigma-1 Receptor Activation:** DMT acts as an endogenous ligand of sigma-1 receptors, which play a role in protecting brain cells during systemic hypoxia, a condition that can occur during a stroke. Activation of these receptors by DMT may support astrocyte survival and reduce cell death in ischemic environments.[24]

- **Reopening Critical Periods:** As mentioned, psychedelics have been shown to reopen critical periods for neuroplasticity, allowing the brain to form and reorganize connections. This property could be harnessed to improve recovery outcomes in stroke patients.[25]

A bit more on Critical Periods

During the critical period, it's important to give yourself time to reflect and relax. Stay clear of the TV, computer and other distractions during this time. It's prime time for integration follow-up sessions with your facilitator, shaman or provider, and if you enjoy journaling this is an ideal time for that too. Journaling and even sketching your thoughts can give an opportunity for inward reflection and growth. If you feel stuck, try taking a meditative hike to clear your mind, or reach out for coffee and conversation with a trusted friend who has a similar or higher depth of psychedelic experiences to share insights. On occasion, one might seek the insight of a few friends, but I recommend seeing a therapist when you are having more complex, difficult emotions or insights that need to be integrated.

In summary, while preliminary findings are promising, the use of psychedelics like DMT in stroke recovery is still under investigation. Ongoing clinical trials and research studies aim to elucidate their safety, efficacy, and mechanisms of action. As this field evolves, psychedelics show major promise towards enhancing neurorehabilitation strategies for stroke patients, especially when combined with other emerging regenerative medicine therapies.

Chapter 6

Psychedelics Benefits to the Microbiome and the Gut-Brain Connection

As a functional medicine physician, addressing the gut-brain connection and balancing the microbiome has been a cornerstone of my practice for a long time. Dysbiosis (an imbalance of bacteria in the gut) is common, and having reliable microbiome testing has allowed me to help balance and improve patients' gastrointestinal function, while also helping them improve their mood and cognition. It's an easy take-home test that simply involves following instructions to place stool in a few containers and shipping it to the lab. Most charge $300-400, and some insurance plans will cover it. Addressing dysbiosis may involve enhancing prebiotic fiber intake through fermented foods, adding probiotics and/or digestive enzymes.

Sometimes testing displays an overgrowth of bacteria, as in small intestinal bacterial overgrowth (SIBO), other times I might find a pathogenic bacteria, protozoa, or parasite that needs treating. These are typically treated with prescription medications, but in some cases, natural protocols can work too.

More recently, research is suggesting that psychedelics can also help with gut microbiome balancing. While I haven't sent patients to the Amazon for Ayahuasca to treat dysbiosis, I have had some share that their irritable bowel syndrome or gut symptoms improved after a week of ceremonial work. About 15 years ago, I was in a circle with a shaman who claimed he cured his Crohn's disease with Ayahuasca. He continues to take a minimal daily dose, which has kept him in remission. Observational data from my patient population and friends in plant medicine circles have supported the ongoing early research findings suggesting an anti-inflammatory effect through a reduction in pro-inflammatory cytokines which may be occuring. Of course more research is needed, and I'm not recommending that Crohn's be treated with daily Ayahuasca. Emerging research suggests a bidirectional relationship between psychedelics and the gut microbiome, indicating that these substances may positively influence gut health. Conversely, the microbiome may modulate the effects of psychedelics.

Preclinical studies have shown that psychedelics can induce changes in the gut microbiota. For instance, repeated administration of lysergic acid diethylamide (LSD) in mice led to modifications in the composition of their gut bacteria. These changes were associated with alterations in the hippocampal endocannabinoid system and kynurenine pathway, which are linked to social behavior and mood regulation.[1]

Additionally, psilocybin has been found to significantly impact the gut-brain axis via the intestinal microbiome in animal models. These effects are partially dependent on its activation of serotonin receptors, suggesting that some therapeutic outcomes of psilocybin might be mediated through changes in the gut microbiota.[2]

Modulation of Bioavailability (Bioavailability is how well a medication or nutrient is taken up into one's bloodstream):

The gut microbiome may affect the metabolism and availability of psychedelic substances, thereby influencing their potency and therapeutic efficacy. Variations in microbial composition among individuals could explain differences in responses to psychedelic therapies. Many of my patients take proton pump inhibitors or H2 blockers when natural treatment fails to treat their GERD. The microbiome is impacted by acid-blocking therapies, and affects the bioavailability of B-vitamins and other micronutrients. Many experienced psychedelic users will employ a technique known as "lemon tekking" to accelerate absorption, reducing the side effects of nausea often encountered with the raw, dried form of mushrooms. It's also my favorite way to enjoy them. Typically, the raw mushrooms are ground up, then lemon juice is added for 30 minutes to help release the psilocin (active ingredient), followed by optional filtering of the ground-up mushroom and then drinking it as a lemon tea sweetened with honey. In effect, the lemons are acting as a digestive enzyme to accelerate the process. This would likely be helpful for those on acid-blocking PPI (Omeprazole) or H2 (Famotidine) GERD therapy. Some theorize that the process dephosphorylates the psilocybin to create Psilocin.[3,4]

I've had a few patients report that psychedelic effects are slightly delayed with psilocybin and Ayahuasca as a result of being on a PPI. Given their significant GERD (heartburn) they elected to continue it while taking plant medicine, but are often delayed in feeling the effects compared to others in a circle.

Personalizing and balancing your microbiome should help optimize your psychedelic therapy. As we begin to understand an individual's gut microbiota, we can offer more personalized and effective psychedelic treatments through better bioavailability and digestion of plant medicines. As mentioned earlier, we assess the microbiome through a functional medicine laboratory and often find natural ways to improve one's gut balance. As we balance the gut microbiome, we are creating a win/win/win situation: reduced inflammation, improved mood, and better absorption of plant medicine molecules and nutrients.

In summary, the interplay between psychedelics and the gut microbiome represents a novel frontier in neuroscience and psychopharmacology, with the potential to revolutionize approaches to mental health treatment as new research emerges. As noted, it's a two-way street; the microbiome can influence the effects of psychedelics, and psychedelics can affect the microbiome composition. Perhaps some will welcome the needed weight loss that comes with a more balanced microbiome achieved through psilocybin microdosing and comprehensive microbiome testing and balancing.

On a personal level, I've found that microdosing has reduced my appetite and created an aversion to alcohol. I used to drink a beer or two a week before this, and now it averages one a month socially, and I've lost the 10 lbs I needed to take off!

CHAPTER 7

Unlocking the Benefits of Expanded Consciousness and Awakening through Psychedelics

I could write another book or two on this topic, and I'm contemplating writing my next book on "Oneness" related to psychedelic states. The benefits of psychedelics have been profound in all aspects of my life, but particularly in the realms of expanded consciousness. Most importantly, I've found that my sense of compassion, empathy, and love have been amplified not simply to my family and friends, but to all of humanity, the world, and the expansive universe.

In this context, when traveling far into states of oneness and ego dissolution, I've found that I am in a state of universal love for all. I often find myself chanting "I am love" when in these very deep states. The people of the world, both good or evil, are loved, and the animals, plants, oceans, mountains, and universe around me are loved down to the deepest level of their subatomic nature, and out to the furthest realms of the cosmos. This has helped me to let go of judging others and to seek to understand them, rather than seeing them as lacking insight etc.

Looking inward, I might have an insight that I need to improve my diet, trust more in the flow of life, communicate better in relationships, and be better at forgiving others or myself.

Many may consider my thoughts to be "Hippy Dippy" or "New Agey", but it is the neuroplasticity and the opening of my consciousness to the multidimensional that has enabled me to see things beyond the pale of our 3D universe. Are the visions I experience on Ayahuasca and other plant medicines mere hallucinations - or are they authentic insights, perhaps even sacred messages, meant to guide my healing and offer wisdom for the betterment of humanity and the Earth?

Most who have travelled several times into the higher dimensions with psychedelics have developed a higher level of nature connectedness, and a desire to preserve nature. Is there an intelligence in psilocybin that is telling us to safeguard a forest so the mycelial network and other mushrooms will survive? Could they have evolved a way to help us recognize that our sustainability and theirs are dependent on preserving nature?

I'm a huge fan of Ram Dass and so wish I could have met him before his passing six years ago. I do feel his presence in the "field" of my plant medicine meditations often, just as I may see Christ, Buddha, and others periodically.

Ram Das was born as Richard Alpert, (April 6, 1931 – December 22, 2019) he was a renowned American spiritual teacher, psychologist, and author best known for his seminal book *Be Here Now* (1971), which became a cornerstone of modern spiritual literature. In his own words, Ram Dass said he'd taken psychedelics "well over 300 times" before traveling to India in 1967. I can only imagine the neuroplasticity and travels to higher consciousness that he experienced with this number of journeys! While in India with his guru he embraced a path of Bhakti Yoga (devotion), blending Eastern spirituality with Western psychology, he became a guru himself significantly transformed by his experiences with LSD.[7] As he combined his expertise in psychology, Hindu philosophy, psychedelic experience, and mindfulness, he has helped many heal and awaken through his teachings.

Religion has unfortunately created division among many across the world. Psychedelics have the potential to soften them for those willing to be open-minded and open-hearted rather than overly judgemental. Simple meditations focused on compassion and oneness can take us to this place as well.

Today, I feel that psychedelics have the potential to break down the rigid walls that are increasingly dividing us. Plant medicines offer a profound path to dissolve the layers of prejudice and bias we've accumulated over decades, allowing us to truly see one another - and to reach out, hand in hand, with unity and compassion.

Have I ever had a "bad trip" or "unpleasant journey"? Well, of course. This has been rare, and usually happened when I have pushed the upper limits on a psychedelic journey, or lacked an ideal set and setting.

While I haven't visualized being eaten by an Anaconda in the Peruvian Amazon during an Ayahuasca journey, I have had a few frightening and unusual journeys to say the least. I integrated these in an open-minded way and have often dissected each scary element within a journey to foster my interpersonal growth and relationship with others and the world. I'm lucky to have friends to integrate with, and when in a group (circle) we typically integrate together the following morning and a week later.

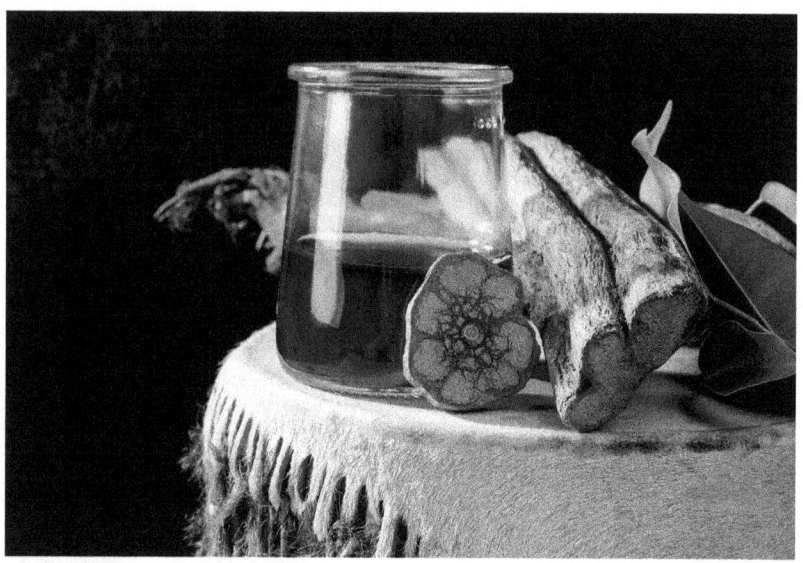

11. Ayahuasca brew, vine and chacruna.

In my 2019 book, "Awakening Gaia, The Lemurian Crystal Grid," I share a true story of an insight that came to me through an Ayahuasca journey, where I was guided to place crystals around the world to balance, honor, and heal Gaia (Mother Earth). While this may sound crazy to many, as one reads the synchronicities discussed in the book, it becomes probable that I may have had insights, or was guided to do this as I connected to a higher consciousness. I feel that most of this work has been done, but I still get an insight that I follow to place another crystal or medicine wheel in various sacred or natural areas. Recently, I placed three crystals in crevices on a coral reef in the Caribbean to help support this struggling ecosystem succumbing to climate change. I'm hopeful others will discover ways to honor our planet in whatever way comes to them, too.

Another book I wrote around the same time, Spiritual Genomics, explores the benefits of sacred geometry, mindfulness, and connecting to nature, as well as other methods for epigenetically shifting your genome to a healthier state. Neither of these books, nor the one you are reading, would have manifested without the enlightenment I've received from psychedelics.

The book idea, chapter outline, and even timeline of writing this book came to me during a psychedelic journey. Writing this particular book has been more scientific, but is fueled by my heart-centered nature of wanting to share knowledge to help others.

So, how have psychedelics changed my brain and others to expand consciousness, heal, and awaken?

Psychedelics alter perception by profoundly influencing brain function, particularly in how sensory information is processed, integrated, and interpreted. Here's a breakdown of the key mechanisms, many of which we have discussed already:

1. Serotonin Receptor Activation (5-HT$_2$A)
- Leads to increased neural activity (fires up your brain in a good way), particularly in the **prefrontal cortex**, which is involved in cognition, perception, and decision-making. The **overactivation of sensory pathways** can cause vivid visual and auditory hallucinations, time distortions, and an altered sense of self.

2. Increased Brain Connectivity

- As psychedelics disrupt normal brain network functioning, particularly the **Default Mode Network (DMN)** it allows for **enhanced cross-talk between brain regions** that don't usually communicate, leading to:

  - **Synesthesia** (blending of senses, e.g., "hearing colors" or "seeing sounds").
  - **Enhanced pattern recognition** (perceiving intricate designs and meaningful connections).
  - **Distortions in spatial awareness and depth perception.**

3. Altered Time Perception

- Psychedelics affect how the brain processes time, often leading to:

  - A **sense of timelessness** (feeling like time has stopped or stretched infinitely).
  - **Time loops or acceleration** (moments feeling longer or shorter than they are).
  - A sense of **living in the present moment without a past or future.**

4. Dissolution of the Ego (Ego Death)

- As they dampen activity in the **Default Mode Network**, psychedelics can reduce the distinction between self and the external world. This can result in:

  - A **sense of unity** with the universe or nature. What I often refer to as "oneness".

- » Loss of **personal identity or boundaries** (also called "ego death").
- » Feelings of deep spiritual or mystical connection.

5. Enhanced Emotional Processing

- **Emotional sensitivity** is enhanced, making experiences feel more pronounced.

- This can bring repressed memories or emotions to the surface, allowing users to process or release held trauma energetically or gain new insights into their psyche. The guidance of a facilitator, who can offer options such as breathwork or energy work, can help in this process.

6. Visual and Auditory Hallucinations

- Common perceptual changes include:
  - » Geometric patterns and fractals overlaying vision are typically more pronounced with eyes closed and/or the use of an eye mask. My favorite is the MindFold mask.
  - » Objects breathing, melting, sometimes becoming more transparent (i.e., looking like you can push your fingers through a granite countertop that appears more fluid).
  - » Enhanced colors, brightness, or vividness. Similar to what photographers refer to as high dynamic range (HDR,) and also seen in the 4K LED TVs. Visual acuity is also improved, with one being able to notice fine detail in the bark of a tree or patterns in a rock.

> Auditory enhancements, noting subtle tonal variations in a violin, the depth of sound in a waterfall, and occasional ethereal sounds. Every note in a musical piece is greatly appreciated in my observations.

7. Mystical or Transcendent Experiences
- Many users report experiences that feel deeply spiritual, including:

    > A sense of infinite knowledge or interconnectedness.

    > Encounters with archetypal figures, divine beings, or otherworldly entities.

    > A feeling of cosmic significance or purpose.

By rewiring how the brain processes sensory input, time, self-awareness, and emotion, psychedelics can dramatically alter perception, often catalyzing profound shifts in consciousness that lead to mystical experiences, heightened creativity, and deep introspection, as I described above. Of course, the intensity and nature of these effects vary depending on the dose, set (mindset), and setting (environment). The neuroplastic benefits of a journey can disrupt habitual thought patterns and help you foster deep introspection. These changes can be temporary or long-lasting, positively impacting your view of the world by:

- **Increasing Openness**: Studies show that psychedelics can increase openness, a key personality trait associated with creativity, curiosity, and willingness to explore new perspectives. Research on psilocybin has found that even a single dose can result in long-term increases in openness, lasting for months or even years. This effect can make individuals more accepting of new ideas, more tolerant of ambiguity, and more willing to engage in deep philosophical or existential reflection.[1]

- **Ego Dissolution and Reduced Self-Centeredness:** As mentioned in prior chapters, psychedelics can disrupt the Default Mode Network (DMN), which is responsible for self-referential thinking and the ego. Applying higher doses of psychedelics often leads to ego dissolution, where individuals temporarily lose the boundaries between themselves and the external world. This experience usually results in a diminished sense of self-importance, an increased level of compassion and empathy for others, and most importantly, a greater sense of interconnectedness with people, nature, and the universe. Sometimes this can be a bit scary, but trusting in the medicine and having a trip-sitter, facilitator, or therapist at your side during your early travels with psychedelics eases the potential anxiety. Traveling to the state of oneness, love, bliss, and acceptance on psychedelics is the ultimate state of ecstasy in my opinion. One must let go, trust, and open their hearts to the infinite universe. I hope that everyone on this planet can experience this state, whether with psychedelics, breathwork, meditation, or sacred sexuality. Yes, it can be similar to a near-death experience (NDE), but you will return to planet Earth as an enhanced being and with a reduced fear of death.

- **Enhanced Emotional Processing and Trauma Healing:** Psychedelics allow individuals to reprocess past traumas and emotions in a non-judgmental, detached way. If working with a trauma therapist, it can help you let go of these more effectively than going at it alone. MDMA is, of course, profound in facilitating this, but a combination of MDMA and psilocybin can provide even greater depth and healing in a nurturing set and setting. Another profound combination is MDMA and 2-CB. For this reason, MDMA, or MDMA with synergistic molecules for couples therapy, offers a portal of loving open communication to help heal differences in opinion, and sustain relationships. This whole process can also reduce fear and anxiety (especially concerning death or existential concerns). For this reason, psychedelics are being used for those in end-of-life situations related to cancer or chronic disease. Currently, I am working with a patient who has a terminal illness who recognizes their time left on this planet is limited. I've referred them to both a therapist and a shaman who have made huge progress in plant medicine journeys to help them let go of this fear and anxiety and to be at peace with their shortened lifespan. I've played a role in assisting them to integrate the sessions, coordinating specialist care, pain management, and taking care of their other ongoing medical issues. I am hopeful that many other physicians will see the benefits of psychedelic medicine in managing end-of-life care. As mentioned earlier, there are clinical studies, as well as my observations regarding psilocybin benefits for terminal cancer patients. Most of the studies found that psychedelics significantly reduced their fear of death and existential distress. Psychedelics also help shift our focus in priorities from material things we get hung up on in life towards families, relationships, and nature. Many will find greater purpose and passion in life, along with greater emotional resilience. Some who have had a past near-death experience (NDE), have noted similar experiences with DMT and deep dives with other psychedelics. Inhaled DMT can often give the "white light" experience, but lacks the life review that many describe from their NDE.

- **Spiritual Awakening and Mystical Experiences:** Psychedelic experiences often induce mystical states, which are associated with a sense of unity or oneness with the universe. Timelessness and transcendence of ordinary reality to higher-dimensional realms are often noted, as well as profound insights into existence and consciousness. While I am a Christian, I don't consider myself religious. Instead, I consider myself spiritual with an appreciation of all religions and philosophies. When I enter psychedelic states of interdimensional consciousness, I have seen Christ, Buddha, archangels, and others who have simply greeted me with unconditional love. No words, just visual or what I'd consider a telepathic communication of pure love, forgiveness, and light. While I'm not opposed to going to church on occasion, I prefer the unfiltered connectedness to the cosmos and the heavenly beings that surround us. As expected, recent and past studies on psilocybin suggest that these mystical experiences can lead to long-term increases in life satisfaction, purpose, and well-being. Over time, many like me have shifted toward more spiritual and holistic worldviews. I've witnessed many who were atheist or despised religion that are now spiritual and at a minimum, appreciate religion and many of the values that religions or gurus may espouse.

- **Shift in Values and Priorities:** Many report a reevaluation of their life goals and relationships after a psychedelic experience. Common shifts include a reduced focus on material wealth and career status. Most will trend towards interests in personal growth, creativity, altruism, and a deeper appreciation for nature and the environment. Some studies suggest that psychedelic use is associated with increased pro-environmental behaviors and a stronger sense of ecological responsibility.

- **Set and Setting for psychedelic journeys:** One of the most essential elements for therapeutic and consciousness-expanding psychedelic journeys is the set and setting. Set is your mindset going into the journey, and the potential map of where you'd like to travel. Are you feeling contemplative and seeking visionary insights about your past or future? Are you considering whether to maintain your relationship with your partner? Do you seek insights to solve a problem or achieve a scientific breakthrough? Perhaps you need to leave it open and simply let the plant medicine show you what you need to see. Do you feel calm or anxious before starting your journey?

In summary, **"Set"** includes your **mood and emotions** (e.g., anxiety, openness, joy, fear), **Intentions** (e.g., healing trauma, creativity, spiritual growth), **expectations** (both conscious and unconscious), **beliefs, and personality structure.** A positive, clear, and respectful mindset - especially one grounded in intention and trust - tends to lead to more beneficial and healing outcomes.

"Setting" is the place where you are experiencing the psychedelic session. This could be an isolated mountain meadow on a summer day, a cozy bedroom with your lover, or a Maloca (ceremonial hut) in an Amazonian jungle with 10 other participants and a couple of shamans. Perhaps you'd like to hike amongst the Native American ruins of Chaco Canyon in New Mexico to connect more deeply to the ancient, enigmatic energies there. For others, it may be lying down on a therapist's office couch while they help you process a trauma. The settings are infinite, but in general, they should foster a calming, safe, secure, and nurturing environment so that one can comfortably let go into the medicine.

Music is often a major part of a healing setting as well, and I can't place enough emphasis on this. Creating or having a friend share a healing playlist for psychedelic journeys is vital to creating a more relaxing setting, and it also engages your brain into a more multidimensional experience that allows one to see enhanced geometry, improved insights, and emotional processing. Sharing playlists from Spotify is encouraged. Of course, if you are in nature, let the sound of a mountain stream, the wind, and birds be your melody. Some light background music in nature can be nice too, but let nature provide the primary auditory stimulus. Again, one has to be able to trust in the medicine, the process, and those around you to find healing or enlightenment. Having an experienced and trusted facilitator or shaman is critical for those beginning to use plant medicines or man-made psychedelics. Facilitators must be safely vetted by assessment of their training, experiences, certifications, reputation, track record, recommendations, etc. Of course, this can often be difficult, especially if going to a retreat in the rainforest, but for many, legitimate reviews and recommendations can be found. Typically, non-profit organizations that aim to promote centers with excellent healing records will list them. If you are doing Ketamine therapy, it should be with a Ketamine trained/certified provider. Now in Colorado and Oregon, you can seek certified and trained psilocybin providers as well.

CHAPTER 8

Synergistic Therapies for Brain Health

One of the most important things we can do for brain health is exercise! Exercise boosts neuroplasticity and neurogenesis. It does this by stimulating BDNF (Brain-Derived Neurotrophic Factor), which supports the growth and survival of new neurons, especially in the hippocampus (crucial for memory and learning). This also helps encourage synaptic plasticity, helping the brain rewire itself for better cognition and resilience.

Key Brain Benefits of Aerobic Exercise

Aerobic exercise enhances hippocampal volume, directly improving short- and long-term memory. Running, swimming, and cycling are great modalities to consider. High-intensity interval training (HIIT) via running or cycling is an excellent option. I enjoy doing a quick 10-15 minute HIIT on an elliptical using EWOT (Exercise with oxygen therapy). It involves breathing high-concentration oxygen (typically 90–95%) through a mask over your mouth and nose during a cardio workout. In doing so, more oxygen is delivered to the brain, further boosting mitochondrial function and BDNF levels. This gives me a chance to push myself a little faster and to end with a nice endorphin rush.

For about $2,000, you can set up EWOT in your home gym. Not cheap, but something to consider if you have the means.

Keeping the hippocampus happy with exercise helps with three types of memory. This includes episodic memory, which allows you to recall personal events and experiences, declarative memory, which enables you to remember facts and knowledge that you can consciously recall, and spatial memory, which allows you to navigate to home or work without relying on Google Maps.

Key Brain Benefits of Resistance Training
Resistance training (also called strength training or weightlifting) plays an influential and often underappreciated role in improving brain health across multiple domains - from memory and cognition to mood and neuroprotection.

Like aerobic exercise, pumping iron can increase BDNF, particularly in older adults, promoting the growth and survival of neurons. In doing so, executive function and working memory are enhanced. Improvements are robust in the prefrontal cortex and hippocampus, regions involved in cognition and memory. Resistance work also reduces inflammation and oxidative stress by reducing pro-inflammatory cytokines and boosting antioxidant defenses, thus potentially reducing your risk of Alzheimer's.

Resistance work also increases dopamine, serotonin, and endorphin levels, improving mood and reducing symptoms of depression and anxiety. It also helps regulate the HPA axis (hypothalamic-pituitary-adrenal axis) activity, lowering chronic stress responses. This keeps your cortisol levels in a more normal range. High cortisol levels can bump up your glucose levels, leading to weight gain and other adverse effects. Prolonged stress may also increase your risk of diabetes by impacting cortisol levels and weight gain, resulting in a negative feedback loop (Figure 12).

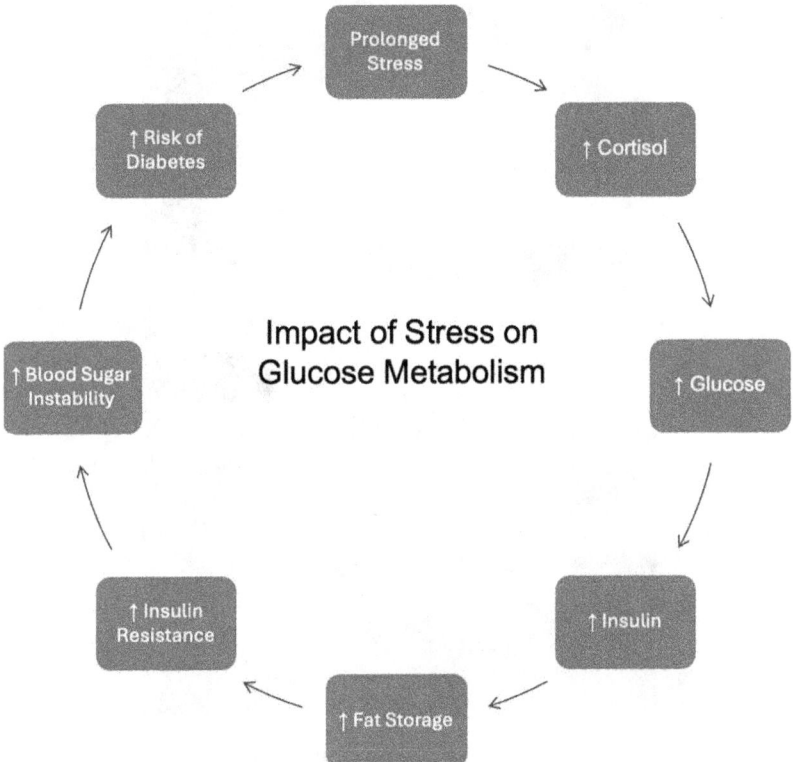

12. Impact of Prolonged Stress influencing Glucose Metabolism

Insulin resistance (metabolic syndrome, diabetes) is a significant risk factor for cognitive decline. As you reduce insulin resistance and improve your glucose metabolism in the brain and body, through aerobic and resistance work, you will lower the risk of type 2 diabetes-associated dementia. As one would expect, resistance exercise also enhances blood flow and oxygen delivery to the brain, which is critical for cognitive function.

Regular strength training has been linked to preserved gray matter volume and reduced brain atrophy (shrinkage) in aging adults. So working out keeps your brain pumped up too.[1,2]

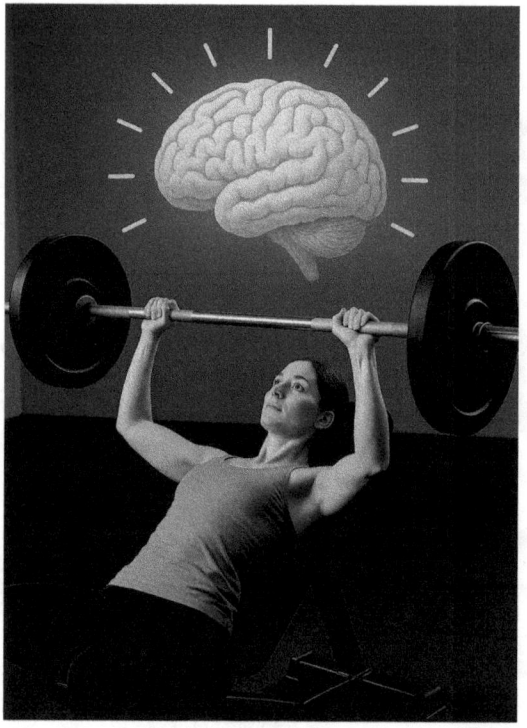

13. Pumping iron can pump your brain!

Balancing hormones to improve physical and mental health

A significant part of my medical practice includes longevity medicine. Often, I encounter patients who are overweight, stressed out, and exercising minimally. As part of my initial panel, I check metabolic markers (A1c, glucose, serum insulin), Growth Hormone level (IGF-1), sex hormones, and inflammatory markers to get a baseline and initial actionable items to identify opportunities for improving their physical and mental health.

Growth hormone and sex hormones can help with neural regeneration and neurotransmitter balance. Testosterone helps with dopamine production, which improves brain speed and can reduce brain fog in those who are low. Testosterone levels are also checked and balanced in women. Estrogen balance modulates serotonin balance, and progesterone enhances GABA activity, which promotes relaxation and better sleep. Balancing all of these can improve mood, reduce anxiety, and give you more passion in life! As I balance hormones in patients, they become more energized, motivating them to show up at the gym or to take that morning run.

Resistance training for brain health should be done two to three times per week and can include: compound movements (squats, deadlifts, rows), bodyweight, and resistance bands.

One should work up to an intensity that is moderate to vigorous, based on individual exercise tolerance. Progress to a gradual overload to stimulate adaptation and strength. Of course, consult your physician on the safety of your workout regimen if you have cardiovascular risk factors. Resistance training doesn't just build muscle - it helps build and preserve the brain, especially as we age.

What about yoga, Tai Chi, and Qi Gong? This form of exercise should also be included in your regimen to help more with balance, flexibility, stress reduction, and mindfulness. If it doesn't fit your style, then look for other forms of exercise that offer similar benefits. Even a hike in the woods listening to a meditation is excellent for the mind and body.

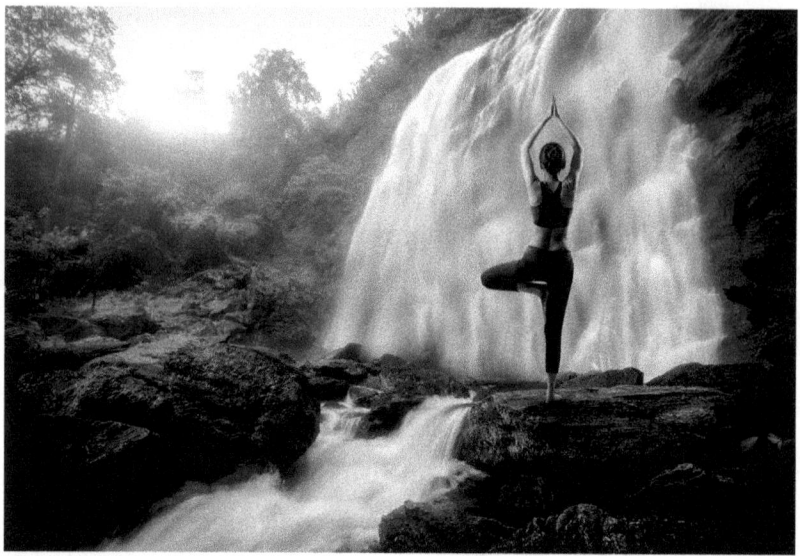

14. Being in Flow with Nature

In summary, exercise is a vital, science-backed pillar of any cognitive longevity strategy. It promotes executive function: decision-making, attention, and problem-solving.

Other benefits of exercise include a reduction in your risk of neurodegenerative diseases such as Parkinson's, Alzheimer's, and other forms of dementia. Amyloid plaque accumulation is reduced, as well as inflammation. In doing so, your sleep, mood, emotional regulation, focus, and cognitive performance will improve. What drug can outdo a robust exercise regimen?

A great, but shocking therapy to consider after a workout is cold water immersion or cold plunge therapy. I have to admit that it's not my jam personally. Having jumped in mountain lakes frequently as a teen on long backpacking trips, I must have gotten that out of my system. I have several of my hardcore friends who swear by it and even seem to seek an identity with it, like marathon runners talking about their last event at a party.

That being said, studies regarding cold water immersion therapy benefits are controversial, and more research is needed. For now, I prefer the mineral hot springs over freezing my butt off, especially after a January powder ski day! Research for cold water immersion has shown dramatic boosts in norepinephrine (up to 2–3x) and dopamine (up to 2.5x) in the brain. This may help improve focus, alertness, and motivation. Some propose that it may enhance mood and one's resilience to depression.[3]

Cold therapy can also activate cold shock proteins (like RBM3), supporting synaptic regeneration and brain repair. Cold stress enhances mitochondrial density and function, which improves ATP production, supporting better brain energy metabolism.[4]

You can set yourself up cheaply by buying a cattle trough for $150, but if you seek a fancy electric cooling tub, plan on spending $2500 to $15,000. Or you can just visit a mountain lake and take a swim! Ideally, one should consider doing this therapy 3–5 times per week at a temperature of 45–55°F (7–13°C) for a duration of 2–5 minutes (gradually build tolerance). Timing is best in the morning or post-workout (avoid close to bedtime).

Optimizing your diet for Brain Health

Pursuing a more ketogenic diet may help reduce neural inflammation. One of my favorites to recommend was developed by Dale Bredesen MD. It's best viewed in his: "The End of Alzheimer's Program: The First Protocol to Enhance Cognition and Reverse Decline at Any Age" It's a comprehensive guide that includes the KetoFlex 12/3 diet etc. Trials supporting a ketogenic diet for brain health are limited, but do show promise and may be worth trying. More research is needed to confirm his and others who claim benefits.

An idea I've considered from a "personalized medicine perspective" is to first get a baseline GFAP level (Glial Fibrillary Acidic Protein Level) and if elevated, initiate a desired brain health diet, then recheck GFAP in 3-6 months to confirm reduction in neural inflammation along with MoCA test or subjective assessments from family members. If markers aren't moving in a positive direction, then reassess and perhaps change the patient's diet to Mediterranean or other, and consider new interventions. GFAP and other inflammatory markers could also be assessed to monitor the reduction in inflammation from psilocybin and other interventions.

Key principles of his KetoFlex 12/3 brain health diet include: **Intermittent Fasting,** where you'll maintain a 12-hour overnight fast (No caloric intake for 12 hours between dinner and breakfast) and a 3-hour pre-bed fast (Finish eating at least 3 hours before bedtime to enhance autophagy and insulin sensitivity.) This encourages a state of **mild ketosis** to provide alternative energy sources (ketones) for the brain, which may be beneficial in Alzheimer's disease due to impaired glucose metabolism. A **plant-rich**, nutrient-dense diet with non-starchy vegetables, healthy fats (extra virgin olive oil, avocados, nuts, and seeds) clean proteins: prioritize wild-caught fish (e.g., salmon, mackerel), pasture-raised eggs, and lean meats.

Promoting a **balanced gut** (microbiome) by including prebiotic and probiotic foods such as asparagus, jicama, kimchi, pickled beets, and sauerkraut is recommended. Inflammatory foods should be limited or eliminated by cutting out added sugars, refined carbohydrates, and processed foods.

Cardiovascular impacts, especially with keto and high-fat diets, should be monitored though, as some may be adversely impacted by bumps in cardiovascular blood markers or find more plaque in their hearts in a follow-up scan on these diets. However, in most cases, this doesn't happen, especially when healthy fats are selected. I check patients' expanded lipid profiles, hs-CRP, uric acid, serum insulin, and A1c, before and two months after initiating ketogenic diets. In patients at higher risk for heart disease, I recommend the Cleerly Heart scan which gives much more detail than the more basic Coronary Calcium Score. Some of my patients experience fatigue and achiness due to lipolysis (breakdown of fat) and the release of toxins. Taking NAC (N-acetyl Cysteine), drinking plenty of water, and promoting lymphatic flow via near infrared light therapy, sauna therapy, and PEMF (Pulsed electromagnetic field therapy) can help accelerate this detox process.

The MIND (Mediterranean Intervention for Neurodegenerative Delay) diet is also recommended for brain health. Researchers conducted a study in which participants were asked to report their diets (Mediterranean versus a diet high in red meat, sugar, and fat). The brains of the subjects were analyzed post-mortem, and the group who had a diet closely aligned with the MIND diet had measurably fewer amyloid plaques.[5]

The MIND diet is similar to the KetoFlex diet, but stresses vegetables, especially green leafy vegetables such as spinach, romaine lettuce, and kale. Also recommended are berries, beans, seeds, nuts, and one or more weekly servings of fish. Eat healthy fats such as avocados and olive oil, while limiting red meat, sugar, and processed foods.

Mindfulness-based activities

The book "Spiritual Genomics" which I wrote back in 2019 discusses the benefits of meditation, sound healing, yoga, dance, breathwork, nature, and other mindfulness-based modalities. In this 400-page book, I share research demonstrating evidence of epigenetic expression as we shift our mind and body to a healthier state through these activities. Many think of mindfulness primarily as meditation, but a hike in nature, appreciating the beauty of a cascading waterfall and the surrounding lush vegetation also counts. As mentioned earlier, I've found that a low dose of psilocybin (for me: 500-1000mg) can tap me into nature, especially by improving pattern recognition of the Fibonacci sequence found in certain flowers (asters), pinecones, and ferns, and even fractal geometry found in corals. In my opinion, this drops us into an even deeper state of mindfulness with an even greater opportunity for healthy epigenetic shifts.

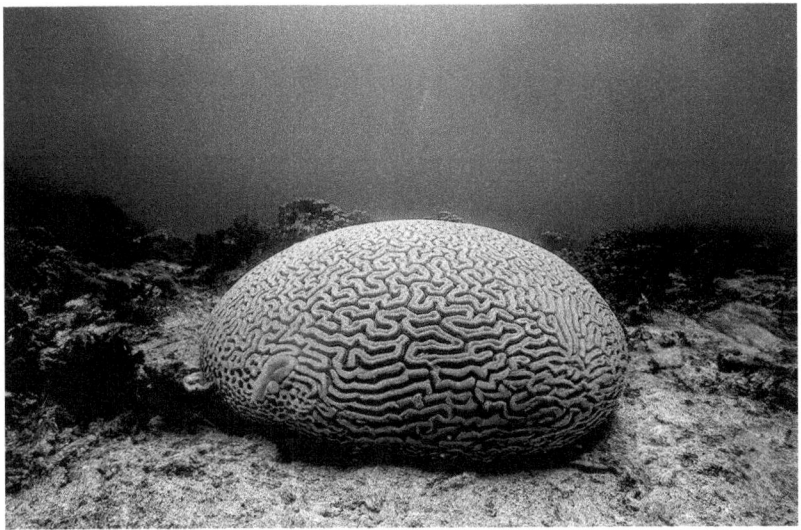

15. Fractal Geometry in Brain Coral

What is Epigenetics? It's the study of changes in gene expression that doesn't involve alterations to the DNA sequence itself, but affects how genes are turned on or off. These changes can be influenced by environmental factors, lifestyle, mind-body balance, diet, stress, and toxins - changes that may even be passed on to future generations.

While I share all sorts of ideas for mindfulness-based activities for my patients, I feel it's best for them to decide what resonates the most with them so that the sustainability of practice is enhanced. For me, it's all about diversity of experiences. While I love yoga, I also enjoy simple nature hikes, fly-fishing, paddling a river, sound healing with crystal bowls, playing didgeridoo or drumming, meditation, and psilocybin journeys with friends. Sometimes I need breathwork sessions to clear my mind of the chaos and turmoil I witness in the world and in our country. If more profound clearing is necessary, I'm often called to Peru to work with Ayahuasca. I remain open and in flow to new experiences and adventurous retreats that come my way too!

Sex and Brain Health

Oxytocin is a significant player in brain health and longevity. Often called the "love hormone" or "bonding molecule" - it's a neuropeptide with powerful effects on the brain and nervous system. While it's best known for its role in social bonding, childbirth, and lactation, research shows it has significant neuroprotective, anti-inflammatory and cognitive benefits. What boosts oxytocin most you may ask? Sex - even more than breastfeeding, but petting your dog, receiving or giving hugs, also helps increase oxytocin.

Oxytocin also helps reduce stress, stimulates neuroplasticity, improves memory (by improving hippocampal function) and has therapeutic potential in the treatment of trauma, neurodegenerative disease, and emotional regulation. It is being researched for its benefits in treating Autism spectrum disorder, PTSD and complex trauma, depression and anxiety, dementia and age-related cognitive decline, and substance abuse recovery (via improved connection and trust). The most profound natural booster of oxytocin is noted post orgasm, and an equal boost is found with MDMA administration.[6]

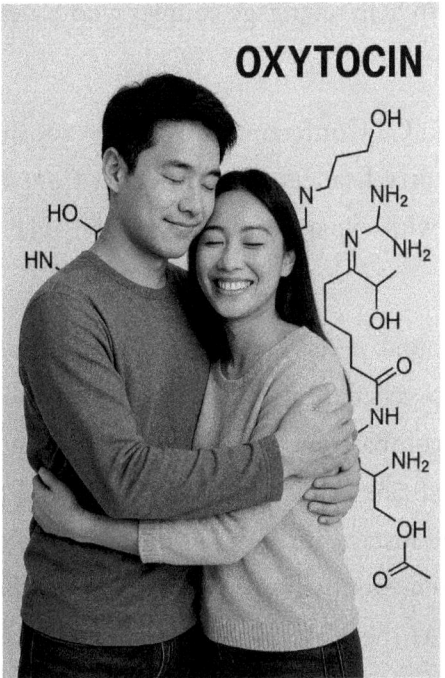

16. Hugs can help release oxytocin!

Oxytocin levels can rise dramatically three to five times from baseline following sex for both men and women!! Emotional bonding, trust, and euphoria are appreciated by most of us following orgasms. Dopamine and prolactin are also released, reinforcing pleasure and bonding post climax.

The boost in oxytocin in a couple enjoying an MDMA journey with music, dancing, body work, foreplay, followed by making love together has not been recorded to my knowledge, but I'd imagine it is close to a 10x bump compared to baseline! A true prescription for love and happiness. We can only hope for MDMA legalization shortly, and perhaps the ability of physicians and therapists to prescribe it appropriately for marital discord, or preventatively to help re-engage couples who have lost their spark for one another.

Perhaps the next G7 Conference (meeting of key European/Asian/American Country Leaders) would benefit from an MDMA session together, with expansion into the UN! (Ha! In my deepest of dreams...)

The most profound transformation I've seen in so many entering the world of psychedelics is their transformation to becoming more loving, compassionate and empathetic human beings. It truly is the medicine to transform the world and make it less divided and more sustainable. It helps individuals go inward to heal themselves, then eventually outward to heal others in a heart-centered way. As they "awaken" to this higher realm, greater insights for transformation can happen. Perhaps an "aha" moment for a unique and collaborative way to solve the worldwide coral bleaching events related to climate change. Or maybe a way to help others find happiness by helping them awaken to the more profound beauty of the surrounding multi-dimensional universe, beyond our messy 3D world.

In regards to MDMA and the oxytocin release, from my own experience and that of others, it creates the most profound state of love, bliss, and heart openness that one can experience. The only thing that I can reflect on in my life that equals this is holding my daughter and son to my heart after each of them was born. I'm sure this is even more the case for mothers.

A growing trend for experienced psychedelic users has been to combine psilocybin or LSD with MDMA and love making, which also increases BDNF dramatically. So while some may frown on enjoying sex and psychedelics, those who are veterans to psychedelics (psychonauts) may actually be robustly enhancing their brain health, relationships and happiness! I'd call this psychedelic relationship biohacking - heart opening while having a mind-expanding psychedelic experience. It doesn't get much better than this. This should only be considered in those with extensive experience and a trusted relationship, and one should always be aware of legal restrictions in your location.

A recent publication and great read titled "Psychedelic Sacred Sexuality" by Astraeus Amori, actually dives into how couples can safely apply psychedelics to enhance the depth of their intimate relationships. The author emphasizes the importance of a safe set and setting with your trusted, consenting lover, while detailing the passionate and tantric states one may experience while enjoying psilocybin, LSD, MDMA, 2-CB, and other potent entheogenic compounds. Drug-plant medicine interaction tables are also included. Opportunities to deepen relationships or heal over issues through a more heartfelt, loving connection (especially with MDMA) abound in this realm.

To summarize oxytocin, I'll share this quote by Ram Dass, "**Love is the most transformative medicine for the soul.**"... and perhaps for the mind and body too.

Sleep and Brain Health

Optimal sleep is critical for brain health. Many of us are unknowingly suffering from sleep apnea, especially those with central sleep apnea, where snoring is typically not present. For anyone who has fatigue during the day, or has any signs of symptoms of sleep apnea, I order a sleep study. It's a good idea to complete the Epsworth and Berlin questionnaires, which are available online, and use the "Snore Lab" app to record snoring, as this can help flag obstructive sleep apnea. Some of my patients prefer to monitor things on their own with smart wearable devices. If you already have a smart watch or ring it's a great idea to keep an eye on your oxygen saturations visible from data transferred to your phone. Most smartwatches and rings do a reasonable job, but often lack continuous pulse oximeter monitoring. So a report displaying that your average oxygen level was 95, won't tell you that you dropped to the 70s several times last night. However, some of the newer rings are starting to offer continuous pulse ox graphs. Another option is to order a constant pulse ox monitor online. These are reasonable at $150-200 and a great home health monitor to have on hand, as well as a blood pressure monitor. No prescription is needed for these. If your levels are below 90 frequently, please bring this to the attention of your physician for a more formal home sleep study to confirm sleep apnea and to determine the best treatment for you.

There are three types of sleep apnea: central, obstructive and complex sleep apnea syndrome. **Central sleep apnea** is a sleep disorder in which the brain temporarily fails to send proper signals to the muscles that control breathing. Unlike obstructive sleep apnea, where the airway is physically blocked, central sleep apnea involves a communication problem between the brain and the respiratory system. This results in repeated pauses in breathing during sleep, often without the usual snoring. Certain medications, such as opioids and benzodiazepines, can contribute to central sleep apnea too.

Obstructive sleep apnea (OSA) is a common sleep disorder where the airway becomes partially or completely blocked during sleep, usually due to the relaxation of throat muscles. This blockage causes repeated breathing pauses, often followed by gasping, choking, or loud snoring. These interruptions can occur dozens or even hundreds of times per night, disrupting normal sleep cycles and reducing oxygen levels in the blood. It's more common in individuals who are overweight, have large necks, or structural airway issues. Having alcohol in the evening can increase OSA events significantly, and medications such as opioids, benzodiazepines, sedatives (Ambien), and barbiturates can make it worse too.

Sleep apnea harms brain health by repeatedly lowering oxygen levels during sleep, which can damage neurons and shrink brain regions like the hippocampus. It disrupts deep sleep, reducing memory consolidation and neuroplasticity. The condition also triggers inflammation and oxidative stress, accelerating neurodegeneration. Additionally, sleep apnea impairs the brain's ability to clear waste products like beta-amyloid, potentially increasing the risk of Alzheimer's disease. Together, these effects contribute to memory problems, mood changes, and long-term cognitive decline. Both types of sleep apnea are linked to daytime fatigue, poor concentration, high blood pressure, and increased risk of heart disease and stroke. Some individuals experience a *mixed form* of sleep apnea, where a single breathing event begins as central (with no respiratory effort) and transitions into obstructive (with effort but blocked airflow). In contrast, **Complex Sleep Apnea Syndrome** is a broader diagnosis that arises when a patient with primarily obstructive sleep apnea develops persistent central apneas during treatment with CPAP or another positive airway pressure device. While both conditions involve central and obstructive elements, mixed apnea describes the nature of individual events, whereas complex sleep apnea reflects a treatment-emergent syndrome affecting the overall sleep pattern. Sleep medicine specialists can help identify the type of sleep apnea you have and guide you toward the most effective treatment. Especially in more complex cases where central and obstructive patterns overlap or emerge during therapy.

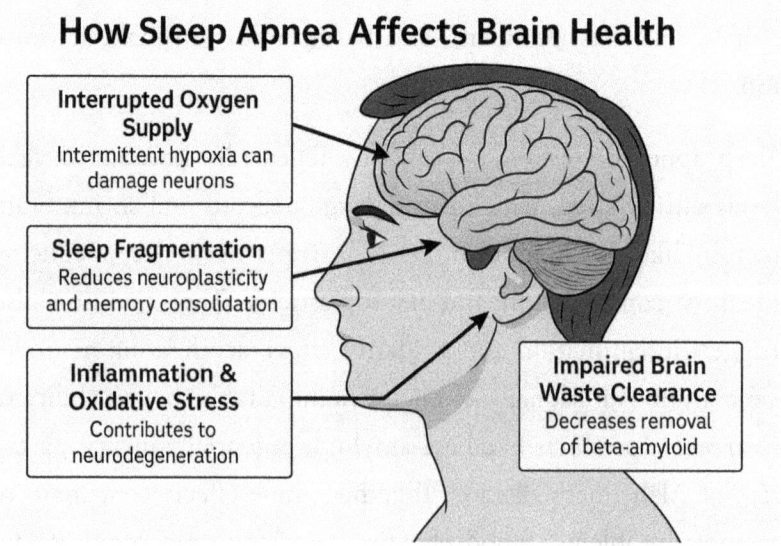

17. The impact of sleep apnea on the brain

Treatment for obstructive sleep apnea (OSA) typically includes continuous positive airway pressure (CPAP) therapy, which keeps the airway open during sleep. Other options include oral appliances (mouthpiece), weight loss, positional therapy, and in some cases, surgery to remove airway obstructions. Another option is the Inspire device, an FDA-approved implantable treatment for obstructive sleep apnea that stimulates the hypoglossal nerve to keep the airway open during sleep. It's an alternative for patients who can't tolerate CPAP, delivering gentle electrical pulses to prevent tongue collapse. The device is controlled by a small remote and works automatically while the patient sleeps. It's an excellent option for those who can't tolerate or respond well to CPAP, but it takes an act of Congress to get approved by insurance due to cost.

For central sleep apnea (CSA), treatment depends on the underlying cause and may include adaptive servo-ventilation (ASV), CPAP, or supplemental oxygen. In cases related to heart failure or opioid use, addressing those conditions is crucial. Certain medications or devices, like phrenic nerve stimulators, may also be used in more complex CSA cases. Other implantable, FDA-approved pacemaker-like devices treat moderate to severe central sleep apnea (CSA) by stimulating the phrenic nerve, which controls the diaphragm. Implanted in the chest, it sends timed electrical pulses during sleep to restore normal breathing rhythms. It's also a tough one to get approved.

My recommendation is to get tested formally with your provider, or at least by home monitoring if you have the slightest concern. In addition to brain and cardiovascular benefits, you'll find that your growth hormones, sex hormones, and thyroid hormones will often improve by treating sleep apnea. This, along with enhanced energy, can help you lose weight if needed and be more productive throughout the day. It's easy to detect and treat, and it can be one of the most important things you can do to help prevent cognitive decline and protect your heart. Oftentimes, a simple oral appliance will work well in milder cases of OSA.

Hearing loss increases the risk of dementia by adding cognitive strain, reducing social interaction, and accelerating brain atrophy, especially in areas tied to memory and language. The brain works harder to process sound, leaving fewer resources for thinking and memory, while social isolation from hearing difficulties further weakens cognitive networks. Studies show older adults with hearing loss are up to five times more likely to develop dementia, but early treatment with hearing aids may help reduce this risk. Bottom line - test your hearing and get it treated early. Online hearing tests are available, but it's best to see an audiologist.

CHAPTER 9

Regenerative Medicine Therapies

Psychedelics, pharmacotherapy or any intervention should always be seen holistically, beyond the context of monotherapy and expanded into a global vision of potential beneficial synergies.

Studying ecology back in my undergraduate years, I appreciated how complex ecosystems are within the varied biomes of nature. An example is the mycelial network of a Pacific Northwest temperate rainforest, a complex interactive system that breaks down leaf litter and other organic matter on the forest floor.

The complex neural network of the human brain resembles a mycelial network, as mentioned earlier in Chapter 1. While we need to study the solitary impacts of LSD on the neural networks of the brain, we also need to examine its interplay with nootropics, mTOR inhibitors, peptides, and hormones to identify synergies that could further improve human cognition, neuroplasticity, and reduce neural inflammation. Ongoing studies using artificial intelligence will be helpful to interpret these very complex interactions.

The field of regenerative medicine offers promising potential to enhance the efficacy of psychedelics and vice versa. For example, stem cell therapy after TBI with psychedelic therapy to stimulate BDNF. Unfortunately, in our extremely subspecialized world of medicine, it's difficult to bring these various disciplines together. Many subspecialists are unaware of regenerative medicine therapies as they are focused on the more traditional allopathic approaches. In my 30-plus years of practice in Regenerative Medicine, I've not yet seen a meeting that would bring us together with psychedelic neuroscientists to brainstorm therapeutic ideas. I'm hopeful to see opportunities for this collaboration in the future.

I'm concerned about limited collaboration amongst academic institutions, as well as their lack of interest in working together with non-profit and private organizations. Less collaboration stifles innovation and delays opportunities for therapeutic outcomes. In some ways it reminds me of the missed opportunities of sharing information between the CIA, FBI, and other areas of intelligence that could have prevented 911.[1] Even 10 years later independent oversight bodies like the Government Accountability Office (GAO) raised concerns that key recommendations - particularly around information-sharing, fusion centers, and integrated intelligence systems - remained only partially implemented, warning that the department was still vulnerable and needed stronger management and coordination. Greater collaboration can equal greater opportunities for prevention and treatment of the Alzheimer's public health epidemic. Independent, critical thinking, creative medical minds will unfortunately remain even further below the radar screen for innovative ideas unless their voice or publication magically goes viral.

I'm hopeful that my words, and those of many others, will inspire deeper collaboration and expanded research across the diverse disciplines within psychedelic medicine. Through this collective effort, I envision a growing psychedelic community that continues to elevate health, enhance well-being, and transform the quality of life for countless individuals around the world. The potential for deeper collaboration and dialogue between indigenous shamans and modern neuroscientists inspires me as well. Let's elevate this from good to truly great, by setting egos aside, and forging a powerful alliance where every voice is valued and respected equally. Now, let's dive into another one of my favorite topics!

Regenerative Medicine

So what is Regenerative Medicine, and why is it important to psychedelic medicine? Regenerative Medicine is basically a discipline that seeks to find therapies that help the body heal itself - or directly provides the building blocks to restore function - often going beyond what traditional medicine can achieve. This may include when indicated: balancing sex hormones, peptide or stem cell therapy to stimulate tissue regeneration, mitochondrial optimization, microbiome balancing, nutrition, and other therapies summarized in the chart below. Much of regenerative medicine also overlaps with functional medicine.

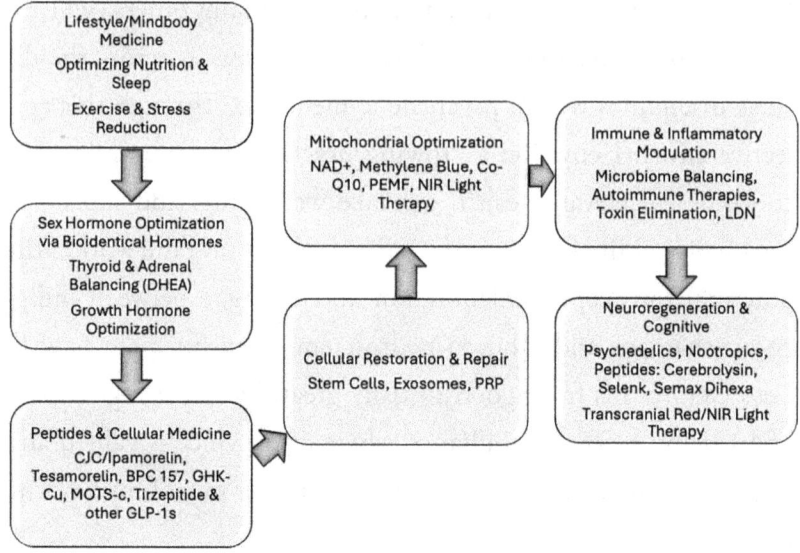

18. Dr. Grover's Regenerative Medicine Algorhythm

Following this basic algorithm, I begin with the basics of nutrition and exercise and then expand into hormone balancing in those who are deficient.

When possible, and if deficiencies and symptoms are noted, I often start early hormone balancing for patients in their late 40s to early 50s. This provides a greater opportunity to take advantage of the profound benefits to the mind and body. The gains from hormone balancing for brain health and prevention of frailty in the elderly are significant. Bone density and reduction in cardiovascular events can be noted for women too.

Of course, HRT should be avoided if there are contraindications such as a history of breast or prostate cancer. However, if the cancer is completely resolved and therapy is cleared by a patient's oncologist, we can consider it cautiously. In those higher-risk patients, more frequent and advanced testing is utilized to monitor them. Oftentimes, I'll use the Galleri screen in addition to traditional mainstream testing for additional reassurance and early detection. See: https://www.galleri.com/. It looks for abnormal DNA patterns shed by cancer cells into the bloodstream, known as circulating tumor DNA (ctDNA).

Standard medical practices check for an average of four to seven types of common cancers: Breast, Cervical, Colorectal, Lung, Prostate, Skin, and Oral cancer. By adding the Galleri blood test for higher-risk patients, we can check for markers of 50 cancers, including pancreatic. I recommend consideration of this blood test for all of my patients over 50 or who have an elevated risk of cancer due to family history or genetic testing.

Balancing estrogen for women may help reduce the risk of Alzheimer's, improve blood flow to the brain, and increase serotonin levels. Brain fog, when present, is often lifted with HRT. In a 2023 meta-analysis covering 6 clinical trials and 45 observational studies, they found that women who received Estrogen-only therapy and combined estrogen-progestogen therapy experienced a **>50 % lower risk of Alzheimer's and other neurodegenerative diseases compared to non-users.** So when your doctor says all hormone replacement is bad, please print up a copy of this meta-analysis and share this data. Greater risk reduction was noted in long-term users (>6 years) versus short-term users (≤ 1 year).[2]

Testosterone in women can help with libido, passion in life, brain speed, post-exercise recovery, and muscle regeneration. Many people, including a lot of more traditional physicians, are completely unaware of the benefits of testosterone replacement in women. In addition to the above, combining testosterone with estrogen also amplifies bone-building benefits. Of course, more orgasms related to increased libido and sensitivy frequently found with testosterone balancing equals greater longevity for both women and men. Several well-conducted longitudinal studies support that more frequent orgasms are associated with significant reductions in mortality risk, making sexual activity a potential contributor to longevity. Smith's 1997 study found that mortality risk was 50% lower in the group with high orgasmic frequency than in the group with low orgasmic frequency, with evidence of a dose-response relationship across the groups.[3,4,5,6]

When I balance hormones for men and women, I assess symptomology via a thorough interview, screen for contraindications, perform a comprehensive exam, and check hormone levels. Women need to be cleared with a normal breast exam and mammogram, and men need to be cleared with a normal psa and prostate exam. Family history is assessed, and if a first-degree relative has a history of early or aggressive breast or prostate cancer, I typically recommend against HRT unless available genetic testing reassures us and the patient is willing to assume the potential risk.

I'm unfortunately seeing many younger men presenting with low testosterone. Symptoms often include low energy, low libido, poor exercise recovery, mid-life crisis symptoms, and depression. I'm now seeing erectile dysfunction for guys in their 30s!! Many experts believe that the earlier onset of low T may be linked to the presence of estrogens in BPA and microplastics. Microplastics have now been identified in human semen, ovarian follicular fluid, and cerebrospinal fluid, indicating their capacity to traverse physiological barriers such as the blood–testis barrier, the blood–follicle barrier, and the blood–brain barrier. These findings suggest potential implications for both reproductive and neurological health, warranting further investigation into their biological effects. Stress and poor diet with minimal exercise, metabolic syndrome (pre-diabetes), or the development of Type 2 diabetes in teens are common contributors as well.

Women are also suffering from earlier onset of perimenopause/menopause, often triggered by metabolic syndrome or Type 2 diabetes, and accompanied by symptoms of low energy, tanked libido, depression, etc.

Taking a functional medicine approach (seeking to address the root cause) I aim first to help women and men reverse diabetes or metabolic syndrome. Oftentimes, this involves counseling them on lifestyle and stress reduction while also coaching them on improving diet and exercise, followed by consideration of GLP-1 therapy such as Mounjaro (Tirzepitide) or Ozembic (Semaglutide). If needed, based on labs and symptoms of menopause or andropause (low T), I'll begin HRT to improve energy and motivation.

My preference for HRT is to utilize bioidentical hormone replacement via topical creams, injectables, or hormone pellets. I avoid old school hormone replacement such as equine-based Premarin and other oral estrogens as they are known to have a higher risk of blood clots. However, oral micronized progesterone is safe. In general, hormone pellets have given the most even-keeled, sustained, physiological balance, with the greatest symptom relief noted by my patients.

Typically, within a few months, major improvements are noted subjectively by the patient, and I usually see improvement in objective observation of blood markers such as A1C's, inflammatory markers, and body composition.

In addition to balancing sex hormones, I'm also addressing thyroid, adrenal and growth hormone imbalances as needed.

Cellular Medicine

Cellular medicine is another major branch of longevity medicine which I offer in my office. This often involves the application of peptides, mitochondrial enhancing molecules, and mTOR therapy as indicated for patients based on their symptoms, labs, age and medical conditions.

Peptide Therapy

The most common peptide I currently prescribe is Tirzepatide for weight weight loss. I may also recommend BPC-157, CJC/Ipamorelin, and Tesamorelin as indicated.

Recent research is suggesting that Tirzepitide (Mounjaro, Zepbound) and other GLP-1 analog peptides may also help in reducing neural inflammation, which may reduce one's risk of Alzheimer's, stroke, and cardiovascular disease. Of course, reversing diabetes with diet and exercise or with a combo of diet/exercise/GLP-1 will also reduce your risk of Alzheimer's.

Many of my biohacking-aligned proactive patients are already requesting that they be prescribed low-dose GLP-1 ("microdose") based on these preliminary beneficial findings. Most are in perfect health with a normal weight and are seeking the potential reduction in Alzheimer's because they have a first-degree relative who was afflicted with the early-onset type. Being a prevention-focused physician, I will prescribe it off-label with the caveat that there are no long-term studies on benefits, and we don't currently know the best dose and duration of therapy. I'm hopeful for long-term studies to determine optimal dosing recommendations in the future. The obvious challenge is waiting 10 years for the results of benefits/risks with GLP-1 and psychedelics being applied preventatively, which may result in a lost opportunity for preventing dementia. There is also a growing interest in microdosing GLP-1 in the general public and hopefully new studies can demonstrate preliminary results at 3-5 years, followed by longer-term studies.[7,8]

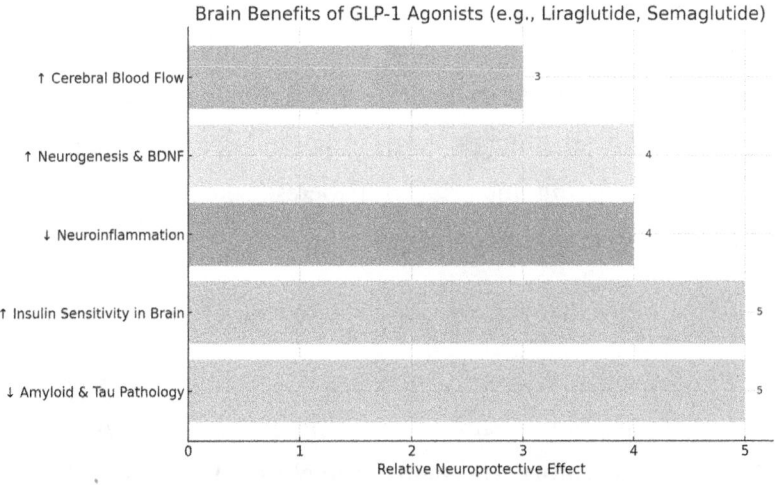

19. GLP-1 Brain benefits based on a review of the current literature.

I use BPC-157 (Body Protection Compound) often in patients to hasten the recovery from tendon or muscle strains, improve soft tissue injury recovery, GI mucosal healing (Crohn's and Ulcerative Colitis, post-GI viral gastroenteritis recovery), brain health, and sexual health via its microvascular blood flow enhancement by nitric oxide (NO) signaling. BPC supports neuroregeneration, the gut-brain axis, and nerve healing. This peptide can be especially helpful post-concussion or for neuroinflammatory conditions. We typically prescribe it as a subcutaneous injection via insulin syringe into belly fat, but we also use oral capsules for inflammatory gastrointestinal conditions.

Tesamorelin and CJC/Ipamorelin are GHRH (Growth Hormone Releasing Hormone) are a few of many analogs that can be used for the treatment of adult growth hormone (GH) deficiency, or in younger individuals who have suffered a traumatic brain injury resulting in low GH levels. Balancing and optimizing growth hormone levels through these types of peptides, or when necessary with growth hormone injections, may also help reduce cognitive impairment and maintain neurotransmitter balance. Positive impacts on the body include maintaining muscle mass and cellular health. The biggest concern is fueling an elusive existing cancer or increasing one's risk of diabetes. Like any intervention, there is a calculated risk.

Other peptides that are more specific to brain health include:

- Semax: a nootropic, increases BDNF, modulates glutamate and dopamine, resulting in enhanced cognition, memory, and neuroprotection, as well as aiding in post-stroke recovery. This is delivered by a nasal spray one to two times per day, and I prescribe it for patients via a reputable compounding pharmacy.

- Selank: another common brain boosting peptide also has anxiolytic benefits (reduces anxiety) by modulating GABA and serotonin. Focus and learning can also be enhanced. It's also a daily nasal spray and can be combined with Semax. I prescribe this one less frequently.

- Dihexa, used to promote synaptogenesis, can enhance memory formation, learning, and may support Alzheimer's therapy. It's experimental, not FDA-approved, but has shown benefits in early animal studies, such as improved maze performance in rats. In neuronal cell cultures, Dihexa increased dendritic spine count nearly threefold and enlarged spine-head width, indicating growth of functional synapses.[9]

- Cerebrolysin: a porcine brain-derived peptide mix that mimics neurotrophic factors (like BDNF, NGF). It is used in stroke recovery, Alzheimer's, TBI, and cognitive decline. It is given IV or IM, typically in a 10–20 day cycle. This peptide is well-studied in Europe and Asia, but is less common in the U.S.

- Thymosin Beta-4 (TB-500): promotes repair, angiogenesis, and neurovascular growth. It may support neuronal recovery post-injury. It's administered by the subcutaneous route weekly and is more beneficial for injury recovery than cognitive enhancement.

Clearing Inflammatory Senescent Cells ("Zombie Cells") via mTOR Inhibition Therapy

Rapamycin (Sirolimus) is the most robust pharmacological intervention known to extend lifespan in mammals. It works through mTOR inhibition, which slows down cellular growth and protein synthesis, mimicking caloric restriction, which is known to extend lifespan. It also enhances autophagy - the cell's cleanup process that removes damaged organelles and proteins. Furthermore, it reduces chronic inflammation and oxidative stress, which are significant contributors to aging. In mice, rapamycin extends lifespan by 10–26%, based on studies by Harrison and Miller. Benefits are noted even when starting later in life, and female animals exhibited a greater extension in healthspan and lifespan compared to males in multiple animal studies.[10] Healthspan is also increased by reducing the incidence of cancer, cardiac dysfunction, and age-related immune decline.[11]

In a 2023 survey of 333 off-label rapamycin users, the researchers noted that the majority of them took it for anti-aging benefits. Respondents stated they felt more youthful, confident, and calm since starting rapamycin.[12] However, this is purely subjective, biomarkers are needed in large human trials to support the anti-aging claims.

Rapamycin's brain health benefits are diverse, exciting, and emerging rapidly! Neuroprotective properties are noted through enhanced autophagy in neurons, which helps prevent the buildup of toxic proteins (e.g., tau, amyloid-beta) in Alzheimer's disease. Neuroinflammation is reduced by inhibiting microglial overactivation, while mitochondrial function is enhanced, and oxidative stress in the brain is also reduced. It may also support neurogenesis in the hippocampus (as discussed earlier), which is critical for multiple forms of memory storage, retrieval, and our ability to find our way back home. So, in addition to lifespan and healthspan benefits, Rapamycin therapy may help improve cognition and reduce amyloid plaques. A 2010 study by Caccamo provides compelling preclinical proof that targeting mTOR with rapamycin may reverse molecular hallmarks of Alzheimer's (amyloid and tau) thus supporting the broader observation that mTOR inhibition improves brain health.[13]

Risks and Considerations

Optimal dosing for anti-aging is not yet determined. Still, most longevity physicians are recommending 6mg once weekly in those who have been cleared of any contraindications, such as a pre-existing cancer. Taking 6mg of Rapamycin before Ketamine therapy or other psychedelic therapy may improve the critical period of metaplasticity and thus offer better therapeutic benefits via a longer-lasting antidepressant effect. In a 2021 study by Zhou, the researchers discovered that it increased the "antidepressant durability" by at least two weeks versus one week without the rapamycin. The authors proposed that this was due to enhanced metaplasticity: the brain was more responsive to future stimuli, not just more plastic in the moment.[14]

As metaplasticity is enhanced, both the stability of long-term memories and flexibility to update or overwrite them is improved.

Declining metaplasticity is linked to cognitive aging and dementia. Enhancing metaplasticity may slow age-related cognitive decline and support recovery from neurodegenerative changes.

Rapamycin is dosed daily for immunosuppression benefits along with other immunosuppressants in transplant patients, which places them at a much higher risk of adverse effects than low-dose once a week for anti-aging benefits. However, as a precaution, I recommend that my patients on a low-dose usage once anti-aging protocol hold their rapamycin if they become sick, are getting a vaccine, or plan to undergo surgery or a procedure. Rarely, potential side effects at low doses may include mouth ulcers, insulin resistance, and lipid changes.

Fisetin is a natural mTOR inhibitor with significantly less potency than Rapamycin, but it is a reasonable and more affordable option to consider. Found in strawberries and apples when concentrated, this natural flavonoid provides a milder, safer, multi-pathway agent that indirectly suppresses mTOR while providing senolytic and antioxidant benefits. It works by activating AMPK, which then downregulates mTOR, giving it senolytic activity. I take capsulated Fisiten a few days out of the week in combination with once a week rapamycin for synergistic and antiinflammatory effects. Eating more lentils, beans, quinoa, nuts, and less red meat or whey protein can also help lower mTOR activity, as well as keeping your diet lower carb with intermittent fasting. As with many longevity strategies, the best diet to pursue for longevity remains controversial, especially when trying to optimize brain health, where a more ketogenic diet is recommended. My approach has been a lower-carb Mediterranean diet.

Mitochondrial cellular support

Ongoing research over the past decade has boosted my ability to optimize mitochondrial health and treat mitochondrial dysfunction. When I first started practicing medicine 30 years ago, all I had in my toolkit was CoQ10 and the recommendation for folks to exercise more or do full-body pulsed electromagnetic field therapy.

CoQ10 or its analogs are always recommended to my patients taking cholesterol-lowering statins to help reduce the risk of muscle aches related to dropping CoQ10 levels and causing mitochondrial dysfunction. Typically, 100-200mg works well, and I recommend it to everyone for additional antioxidant benefits. Ubiquinol, a more bioavailable analog, is better for older adults or those with chronic medical conditions. As our air quality continues to deteriorate due to rising ozone and subsequent oxidative stress, we can mitigate these effects by taking CoQ10 or Ubiquinol and avoiding outdoor runs when the air quality index (AQI) exceeds 60. Wildfires here in the Rocky Mountain West are on the rise with climate change, and each summer I find myself stuck inside sadly when the AQI is 120 or higher. During severe bad-air days, I take at least 200mg of CoQ10 and oral 500mg of S-acetyl glutathione twice daily. When I see folks running on these days I often think it's the equivalent of smoking two packs of cigarettes!

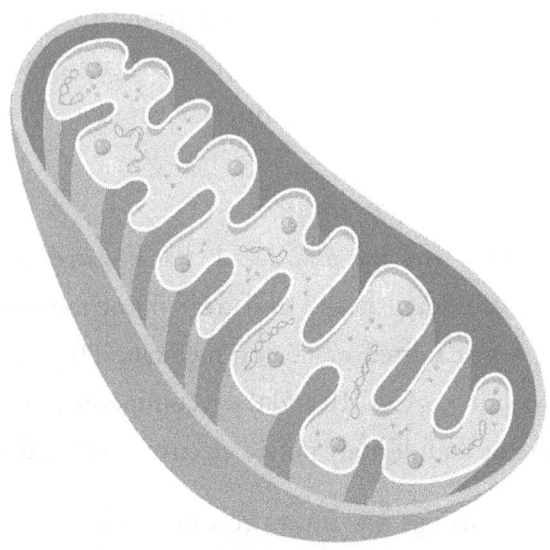

20. Basic Mitochondrial structure

NAD⁺ Therapy (nicotinamide adenine dinucleotide)

In the last 10 years, NAD⁺ has become a very popular functional and regenerative medicine approach to optimizing mitochondrial function and for the treatment of mitochondrial dysfunction. It's also popular amongst psychiatrists who use it to augment the treatment of depression. Intravenous NAD⁺ therapy began back in the 1960s in the United States when it was used primarily to aid in addiction and withdrawal treatment. Over the following decades, it has become more mainstream in helping individuals seeking better energy and mental clarity, aiding overall cellular health and anti-aging, supporting brain function (including neuroprotection), and mood stabilization. How does it work? NAD⁺ improves energy by acting as a central coenzyme in the production of cellular energy (ATP), especially in mitochondria, the "powerhouses" of your cells. Without enough NAD⁺, ATP production slows - leading to fatigue, brain fog, and reduced endurance. While we don't have large randomized trials yet, the response in the majority of patients is dramatic. Many of my patients using Oura rings and smart watches have shared data displaying huge improvements in HRV (heart rate variability), endurance, and post-exercise recovery. Since NAD⁺ is generically available, it is unlikely that a large study will be performed, unless it is patented and monopolized for financial gain. If this occurs, this expensive IV treatment averaging $600 a session, will easily become $2400 or more. In the last decade, we brought NAD⁺ and precursor molecules NMN (Nicotinamide Mononucleotide) and NR (Nicotinamide Riboside) into my clinic to help enhance mitochondrial function for all the beneficial reasons mentioned above. For biochemists, NMN is a direct precursor to NAD⁺ in the salvage pathway. NR is another precursor to NAD⁺, but one step further upstream than NMN. It converts to NMN, then to NAD⁺. Both NMN and NR are more affordable ways to boost your NAD⁺ levels, at least for now…

The FDA's move to ban NMN as a dietary supplement in late 2022 is partly regulatory, but most likely influenced by pharmaceutical financial interests. The FDA then ruled that NMN must be classified as a drug-in-development, not a supplement. Today, this supplement remains in a grey zone of future OTC availability, much like NAC did a couple of years ago. Clearly, a few pharmaceutical companies are seeking to block future affordable access to NMN for their own financial gains as noted by recent and ongoing legal action. NMN products being developed by MetroBiotech, (Co-founder David Sinclair Ph.D) filed an Investigational New Drug (IND) application before NMN was notified as a dietary ingredient. As a result of these legal actions, NMN may be taken off the market in 2025. Elysium, Life Biosciences etc, are also looking to cash in on the hopes of it becoming a prescription medication. While I am grateful for ongoing R&D by Sinclair and others, I feel that basic NMN and NR supplements should remain accessible OTC as more bioavailable analogs with greater potency are reasonable to classify as drugs. In this way, we seek a win/win.

It truly has been a game changer in the treatment of long COVID and associated brain fog and severe fatigue. SARS-CoV-2 (the virus that causes COVID-19 and variants) can impair mitochondrial function, leading to fatigue, brain fog, and poor recovery. Post-COVID fatigue symptoms are related to mitochondrial dysfunction and the depletion of NAD^+. Our clinic and many other functional medicine physicians have noted that replenishing NAD^+ via IV therapy, Subcutaneous injections or oral NMN may help expedite recovery. As we restore NAD^+ levels, cells may regain energy-producing capacity and reduce metabolic dysfunction. Long-COVID is associated with persistent inflammation and immune activation. NAD^+ activates sirtuins (especially SIRT1 and SIRT3), which suppresses pro-inflammatory cytokines, inhibits the NLRP3 inflammasome (a key player in COVID-related inflammation) all while supporting the resolution phase of immune responses. I'm hopeful that the application of NAD^+ may reduce the risk of neurodegenerative disease, especially after a massive inflammatory reaction after catching SARS-CoV-2. Those who have adverse vaccine reactions to the COVID-19 vaccine may also benefit from NAD^+ and glutathione therapy.

NAD⁺ influences neurotransmitter balance, neuronal repair, and neuroplasticity. It also boosts BDNF indirectly via SIRT1, and reduces oxidative stress in the brain, a likely contributor to post-COVID cognitive symptoms. In addition to NAD+ for long-COVID, we often deploy other regenerative peptides such as BPC-157, give IV Glutathione and Vitamin C, and optimize the gut microbiome with probiotics if needed. I've observed most allopathic providers (traditional medicine) managing Long-COVID by simply prescribing an SSRI or SNRI antidepressant rather than seeking to address the root cause which is residual inflammation and mitochondrial dysfunction.

Beyond its use in post-COVID therapy, it has notable benefits for our patients over 40 with age-related cognitive decline, those seeking better cognitive performance, or for those seeking additional support in the reduction of their depressive symptoms.

In my patients with moderate to severe depression who have been prescribed SSRI's or SNRI's, I will often do several IV NAD⁺ sessions at 750mg each and then follow this with several sessions of Ketamine. This combination has been much more effective than using SSRI or SNRI therapy. In addition, many of my patients will start self-microdosing psilocybin for mood maintenance after completing a series of NAD⁺ and Ketamine sessions. Alternatively some may find that a larger, more stimulating, once every one to two months of 2-4 grams of dried psilocybin mushrooms is more effective than microdosing at 100-200mg four days a week.

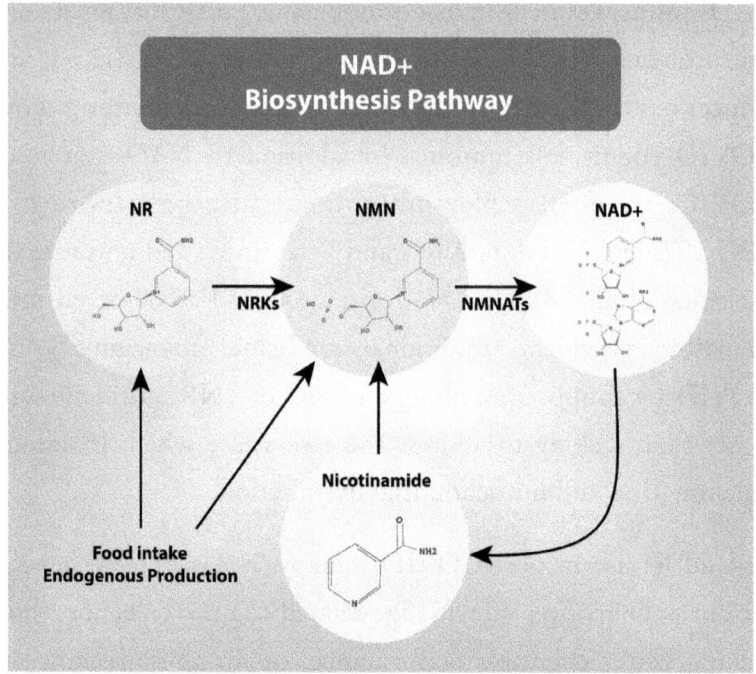

21. NAD⁺ Synthesis

I personally take NAD⁺ 100mg subQ twice weekly, along with a daily NMN supplement. When time allows I do 750mg IV infusions over a two hour drip time. This has helped keep my energy optimal, and has allowed me to work on this book late nights after a full day of seeing patients! Interestingly I've observed an increase in sensitivity/responsiveness to psilocybin journeys, suggesting better neurotransmitter balance and/or receptor responsiveness.

I believe that NAD⁺ may amplify the long-term therapeutic benefits of psychedelics by enhancing the brain's ability to rewire and form lasting emotional and behavioral shifts. This happens as NAD⁺ boosts neuroplasticity via SIRT1 activation (a longevity and plasticity gene), increasing PGC-1α, promoting mitochondrial biogenesis, and the regulation of CREB - a transcription factor linked to memory and synaptic growth. With these benefits in mind, please see the table below for consideration of psychedelic journey/session enhancements.

Dr. G's NAD⁺ Protocol to consider for enhanced effects of a psychedelic session

Timing	Use of NAD⁺	Potential Benefit
Pre-journey (1–3 days)	NAD⁺ 750mg IV, or 100mg sub-q for 3 days prior. Oral NR/NMN at typical doses is a third option.	Boost mitochondrial energy, reduce brain fog
Day of Session	Optional 250mg NAD⁺ IV (low dose) or Sub-Q 100mg is another good option. Oral NR/NMN is another option. (Consider Rapamycin 6mg as mentioned earlier for mTOR benefits)	Enhance clarity, resilience
Post-session (integration phase)	NAD⁺ (low or high dose via oral or IV.) CoQ10 100mg, L-carnitine 1000mg, Magnesium Threonate 500mg and Lions Mane for a week. Methylene Blue 20mg can be started a couple days after journey. Do all these daily for a week.	Support neuroplasticity and cognitive processing

Methylene Blue

Methylene Blue (MB) is another powerful mitochondrial booster, but it works through a different mechanism of action than NAD+. This phenothiazine dye was first synthesized in 1876 by German chemist Heinrich Caro at BASF (Badische Anilin und Soda-Fabrik). Developed initially as a textile dye, methylene blue quickly found applications in medicine, becoming one of the first synthetic drugs. This included the treatment of malaria and the staining of cells for microscopic analysis, helping to lay the groundwork for modern histology and neuroscience.

My first exposure to MB was in my cell biology class in college, followed by using it in histology class at medical school. We typically used it to visualize bacterial size, shape, and arrangement under microscopy. I remember it well because I would occasionally leave the lab with blue fingertips if I wasn't being careful! It's FDA-approved for use in methemoglobinemia (restores hemoglobin's oxygen-carrying capacity), as a urinary tract antiseptic (blocks bacterial growth), and for Malaria (historically). More recently, it's been studied and appreciated for its nootropic, neuroprotective, and mitochondrial benefits at low doses. While some clinicians may be skeptical of MB benefits, I can, without doubt, confirm that the majority of my patients notice improvements within a week at 20mg or higher dose.

How does it work? MB can accept electrons from NADH and donate them to cytochrome c, bypassing damaged portions of complex I or III in the electron transport chain (ETC). This "bypass" helps maintain ATP production even when parts of the ETC are impaired, crucial in aging or neurodegenerative diseases.

Typical dosing for longevity enhancing aimed at improving energy, brain health, and neuroprotection is 0.5–2 mg/kg body weight. I typically start my patients on a lower dose at 20mg/day and then incrementally increase the dose up to 80mg over a few months based on response and whether or not they have a neuroinflammatory condition. For those with Parkinson's, Multiple Sclerosis, or Alzheimer's, I typically bring their dose up to 60-80mg daily. Taking half in the morning and the other half in the afternoon is best when possible.

Here is an example of supplements one might consider for mitochondrial optimization-

Supplement	Typical Dose	Key Function
Methylene Blue	0.5–2 mg/kg daily (max 5 mg)	Electron carrier, ETC support, antioxidant
NAD⁺ precursor (e.g., NMN or NR)	250–500 mg/day	NAD⁺ replenishment, energy metabolism
CoQ10 / Ubiquinol	100–200 mg/day	Electron transport, antioxidant, statin support
Acetyl-L-Carnitine	500–1,000 mg/day	Fatty acid transport into mitochondria
Alpha-Lipoic Acid	300–600 mg/day	Redox cycling, antioxidant, insulin sensitivity

Supplement	Typical Dose	Key Function
Magnesium (glycinate or threonate)	200–400 mg/day	ATP cofactor, NMDA modulation. I use it to help calm myself during a journey if I'm overstimulated. (CBD 30-60mg is also helpful for this)
PQQ (Pyrroloquinoline quinone)	10–20 mg/day	Mitochondrial biogenesis
Resveratrol or Fisetin	100–250 mg/day (cyclic)	SIRT1 activation, inflammation control

Near Infrared Light Therapy and Photobiomodulation

I've been an advocate of NIR light therapy for decades recommending panels, light therapy pads and transcranial NIR light therapy. We have several NIR light therapy pads that we use to reduce muscular inflammation in patients, and we also apply it for photobiomodulation during methylene blue infusions. In 2019, I was a Co-Principal investigator in a study that evaluated transcranial near-infrared light therapy for the treatment of TBI in Veterans. We demonstrated an improvement in neuropsychological scores in 6 of 15 subscales (40.0%; $p < 0.05$; two tailed) and a SPECT analysis displaying an increase in rCBF (Cerebral Blood Flow) in 8 of 12 (66.7%) in study participants.[15]

Activating the methylene blue with near-infrared light (NIR light) at a wavelength of 660–850 nm can truly turbocharge the benefits of MB to the mitochondria since they both stimulate mitochondrial function via the Cytochrome c Oxidase pathway in the electron transport chain. The light increases electron flow, resulting in increased ATP production, increased mitochondrial membrane potential, and a decrease in oxidative stress. When used together, the combination produces a shared mechanism of neuroprotection, acting synergistically to enhance ATP production, reduce oxidative stress, and protect against degeneration.

My preference for patients with cognitive impairment or depression is to use the Vielight transcranial NIR device with intranasal NIR. My current favorite is the Vielight Neuro Pro 2. (You can use a discount code Revmd if you'd like a 10% discount on a Vielight when ordering online.)

Preclinical models show greater increases in ATP levels when MB and NIR are combined vs either alone. One rat brain study suggested up to 30–40% greater ATP production using this combination. Faster Recovery from Brain Injury has been noted with MB + NIR. This combination improved cognitive and motor recovery post-TBI in animal models more effectively than either therapy alone.[16]

Case Example for Alzheimer's Support via MB and NIR Light Therapy

- Take 40 mg methylene blue orally (capsule best)
- Wait 30–45 minutes

- Apply red/NIR light to forehead for 20 minutes (e.g., 810 nm light) I recommend the VieLight or similar transcranial NIR light unit combined with a nasal NIR probe. Repeat daily, or at least 3 times a week.

MB should be avoided with SSRIs, SNRIs, and other serotonergic drugs due to MAOI activity and a slight risk of serotonin syndrome. For this reason, one should also avoid it on the day of a psychedelic session, and it's a good idea to hold it for a couple of days before and after psychedelics. MB should also be avoided in those with G6PD deficiency and in pregnancy. If you are taking a reasonable dose, it should turn your urine blue. This is otherwise harmless, except that the toilet rim may become speckled blue if guys with a sloppy aim are around! Be sure to take a USP grade, pharmaceutical quality MB (non-industrial grade only). I prefer capsules and take 25mg daily myself, but many will opt for the less expensive dropper version. When using the liquid version, be careful with your clothes and squirt it on the back of your tongue.

Could Lithium Prevent or Reverse Alzheimer's Disease?

In a recent ten-year long study just published in Nature, researchers demonstrated how lithium provides protection to the brain by shielding it from neurodegeneration. In the brains of mice with low lithium levels, researchers noted a dramatic increase in amyloid beta deposits and neurofibrillary tangles compared to mice that had normal levels of lithium. According to senior author Bruce Yankner, "The idea that lithium deficiency could be a cause of Alzheimer's disease (AD) is new, and suggests a different therapeutic approach." The authors noted that lithium orotate helped reverse the Alzheimer's pathology, prevented brain cell damage, and helped restore memory in the lab animals.[16] Bottom line, low-dose lithium orotate could be of major therapeutic value in preventing and reversing AD. Human trials will be needed of course, but I'm hopeful to see promising results in the near future once the trials begin.

Pulsed Electromagnetic Field Therapy (PEMF) and Transcranial Magnetic Therapy

Pulsed Electromagnetic Field Therapy (PEMF) increases mitochondrial membrane potential, which is crucial for driving ATP synthase to generate energy. In simpler terms, it charges up your cells' batteries, helping them make more energy. Studies show PEMF can improve the efficiency of the electron transport chain (ETC). As it improves microcirculation and oxygenation of tissues, it then increases the availability of oxygen for oxidative phosphorylation, making mitochondria more efficient at ATP production. PEMF also activates CREB, promoting mitochondrial biogenesis, which enhances synaptic plasticity and repair in neurons. CREB is a transcription factor which is a type of protein that binds to specific DNA sequences to upregulate the expression of certain genes to enhance brain health. CREB can also increase BDNF. Exercise is another great way to increase CREB and BDNF as mentioned earlier.

PEMF therapy leads to more resilient, powered up, and abundant mitochondria in aging or damaged tissues. The number of mitochondria (mitochondrial density) in a muscle cell will increase with PEMF therapy for example. I love this device so much that

I have one at my office and one at home! I sandwich myself between a full body near-infrared panel suspended on a motorized stand a foot above me, and the similar length PEMF mat under my body. This dual therapy of PEMF and NIR is one of the best ways you can power up your mitochondria, especially if you take methylene blue an hour prior.

In a study of bone regeneration using PEMF, Wang found that PEMF can also activate the mTOR signaling pathway, upregulating regenerative proteins, boosting cellular metabolism and viability, indirectly supporting mitochondrial function.[18]

Brain training with Neurofeedback (EEG biofeedback) is a noninvasive brain training technique that teaches individuals to self-regulate their brainwave activity. It supports neuroplasticity by training the brain to self-regulate dysfunctional patterns, promoting more efficient and flexible neural networks. This adaptive rewiring can enhance learning, memory, and emotional resilience. By reducing stress and improving autonomic balance, neurofeedback may also help increase levels of Brain-Derived Neurotrophic Factor (BDNF), a key molecule involved in neuronal growth, repair, and synaptic strengthening. As a result, neurofeedback shows promise in managing a range of brain-related conditions, including anxiety, depression, ADHD, PTSD, autism, and cognitive decline, by enhancing the brain's capacity to reorganize and heal itself. I had a neurofeedback practitioner in my office for five years and observed the benefits of brain training for many of my patients. QEEG brain mapping was performed before and after to monitor improvements, as well as other subjective and objective measurements. It's worth considering, especially since AI integration with neurofeedback is allowing for easier home-based therapy. It's time-consuming in the office and can be cost-prohibitive for some in this setting. Having a certified neurofeedback specialist help you with home therapy and also perform an initial and follow-up brain map is best to optimize outcomes.

Transcranial Magnetic Stimulation (TMS) is a noninvasive neuromodulation technique that uses rapidly pulsed magnetic fields to induce small electric currents in specific brain regions, most commonly the left dorsolateral prefrontal cortex. These currents stimulate or inhibit neural activity, depending on the frequency used, and promote neuroplasticity, synaptic strengthening, and restoration of functional connectivity in mood and cognitive networks. TMS enhances the expression of BDNF, improves cerebral blood flow, and modulates neurotransmitters like serotonin, dopamine, and glutamate. Clinically, TMS is FDA approved for treatment-resistant depression, OCD, and smoking cessation, and shows promise in conditions like PTSD, Alzheimer's, and chronic pain by improving mood, cognition, and emotional regulation without the systemic side effects of medication. I've seen great results with this therapy for my patients with treatment-resistant depression. Insurance coverage can be limited and often requires you to have failed two to three different antidepressants, typically before being covered. 50-70% of treatment-resistant patients respond to therapy, which is impressive.

Transcranial Direct Current Stimulation (tDCS) is a noninvasive neuromodulation technique that applies a low electrical current (typically 1–2 mA) to the scalp to modulate neuronal excitability. Anodal stimulation increases cortical activity, while cathodal stimulation decreases it, allowing targeted enhancement or suppression of brain regions involved in cognition, mood, and motor control. tDCS has been shown to improve working memory, attention, language processing, and mood in both healthy individuals and those with neurological or psychiatric conditions. It is being studied for its potential benefits in depression, stroke rehabilitation, Alzheimer's disease, and age-related cognitive decline, with minimal side effects and a strong safety record with repeated use.[19]

There are consumer-grade tDCS devices available that are generally considered safe when used correctly, but they must be used with care, proper placement, and awareness of contraindications. These devices deliver low-level electrical stimulation (typically 1–2 mA) and are designed for home use to support focus, mood, memory, or recovery. I've had a few computer gamers share that they have used them to improve their reaction times when competing with others online. I typically recommend NIR therapy over tDCS, but share this as an option to patients as well for cognitive enhancement.

Exosome and Stem Cell Therapies are emerging regenerative approaches for brain health, showing promise in conditions like Alzheimer's, traumatic brain injury (TBI), stroke recovery, long COVID, and cognitive decline. Ongoing developments in this field are allowing for more targeted stem cell deliveries, and may even be helpful for age-related hearing loss in the future.[20]

Exosomes are nano-sized vesicles secreted by stem cells that carry growth factors, microRNAs, and anti-inflammatory molecules. They can cross the blood–brain barrier and modulate neuroinflammation, support neuronal repair, and improve synaptic function. Stem cells, especially mesenchymal stem cells (MSCs) derived from umbilical cord, bone marrow, or adipose tissue, offer similar benefits by reducing inflammation, increasing BDNF and NGF levels, and stimulating neurogenesis and mitochondrial repair. While neural stem cells (NSCs) are still largely confined to research, MSC-based therapies are being used off-label in some U.S. clinics and more widely in offshore facilities in Panama, Mexico, and the Cayman Islands.

Although these therapies are not FDA approved for neurological use in the U.S., they are accessible through investigational protocols and at some integrative/regenerative medicine practices. Administration routes include intravenous, intranasal, and (more rarely) intrathecal delivery. We have offered the off-label intranasal use for patients who have lost their sense of smell from COVID-19, and for treatment of TBI and mild cognitive impairment with reasonable success, especially when combined with other complementary therapies. Some of our patients have traveled to Panama to receive stem cell therapy, but this is extremely expensive and out of reach for most financially. I'm still not convinced that this expensive therapy provides ROI at this point at $20,000 or more per treatment.

Ongoing clinical trials and observational data suggest benefits in improving memory, cognition, fatigue, and neuroinflammation. We've noted this as well, especially where combinations of exosomes or stem cells with other regenerative therapies - such as NAD$^+$, red/NIR light therapy, methylene blue, or neuropeptides, may further enhance outcomes by synergistically supporting mitochondrial and synaptic function. As research progresses, these biologics may play a central role in personalized brain regenerative medicine protocols.

I'm hopeful that ongoing research will lead to improved efficacy and safety, providing the data needed for FDA approval. I do feel there's a pushback from big pharma and other medical device companies as they fear a huge loss of profits as stem cell therapies become more targeted and effective, freeing patients from a lifetime of medication or device dependency. Logically, lobbyists from many pharmaceutical companies have, and will continue to invest in making regenerative therapies such as peptide therapy, exosome, and stem cell therapies more difficult to obtain in the U.S. to help preserve their profits. Ongoing restrictions in regenerative medicine therapies in the US will also result in more medical tourism and billions of dollars lost to our economy.

Imagine the impact of improving your health span and quality of life through targeted stem cells, helping to reverse neurodegenerative conditions, hearing loss, renal failure, heart failure, arthritis, and more. The nursing home/long term care industry, hearing aid centers, and joint replacement centers would lose billions while the elderly are able to stay at home and on their feet, avoiding the depleting of their life savings.

According to estimates by the Centers for Medicare & Medicaid Services (CMS) the U.S. spends close to $5 trillion annually on healthcare representing 17.3% of our GDP, compared to European countries that spend on average 9-12%. Moreover, we spend twice as much per capita on health care than most European nations. We are also spending 10-30% of our annual income on healthcare insurance, which is not sustainable with the rising cost of living. Despite higher spending in our country, outcomes for chronic disease, maternal health, and preventable deaths are worse. Something radical needs to change.

I predict that the recent cuts to Medicaid in 2025 will end up costing our system twice as much as saved in the long run by cutting access to preventative care, chronic medical care (i.e. uncontrolled diabetes), resulting in thousands of unnecessary and preventable emergency room visits that will ultimately be paid for by you and me. Cuts to climate monitoring and early detection of severe weather will cost us more in the long run as well. We clearly need to be more proactive in monitoring severe weather events such as flooding, fires, hurricanes and tornadoes and should have more sensors and monitors placed to alert inhabitants immediately.

What is the best thing we can do? In my opinion, all of us must do our best to maintain better health and seek to adopt as many preventative and regenerative medicine strategies to keep ourselves out of the hospital! As a country, we need to address things more preventively and proactively, rather than being reactive and playing the blame game. Much of this requires us to be self-informed on the best health strategies beyond what a ten-minute visit to a primary care office can recommend. Reliable sources are available online, but one must know how to filter through the misinformation provided by social media, Doctor Google or AI. We must do what we can to call out the greed of managed care, big pharma, and unethical lobbying toward Congress aimed at keeping us sick for corporate profits, rather than moving us towards wellness. Yes, they need to make a profit, but it should be done ethically, at a reasonable price, while not superseding lifestyle changes that could reverse a condition safely.

CHAPTER 10

Final Thoughts

Psychedelic medicine offers immense potential for advancing brain health, unlocking new pathways for healing, neuroplasticity, and mental well-being. Much of this depends on our ability to destigmatize, educate the public, and fund research in this area through a multifaceted team-like approach amongst academic institutions, foundations, non-profits, and individuals.

This will require bold, creative, visionary, and collaborative actions of all involved, with reasonable funding from governmental and non-governmental sources to move it forward. International sharing of insights will further accelerate the effort to the extent they are willing to do so.

In addition, going beyond an entrepreneurial mindset seeking philanthropy with sustainability is necessary to move this forward for the advancement of humanity on both cognitive and spiritual levels. Entrepreneurial interests are reasonable for sustainability, but again, they shouldn't be the primary motive for advancing this field. An opportunity for everyone to have access to these therapies should be a core value in honoring the spirit of plant medicine. When we lead and invest in a heart-centered way, we unlock a ripple effect - fueling groundbreaking research and transformative treatments, and sustaining a future where compassion and innovation drive lasting change.

Concurrently, we should inform the general public on the benefits of psychedelics through more scientific, evidence-based findings on their benefits, and contrast them to the harmful nature of alcohol and opioids which are killing thousands annually. While "Burning Man" and other smaller festivals are cool and much needed, they shouldn't be the poster child for the psychedelic renaissance. An emphasis on treating addiction through psychedelics and more effectively treating mental health issues is needed.

Many plant medicines have been used for thousands of years by shamans in cultures around the world with success. We need modern-day shamans who will respectfully integrate the knowledge and shared expertise of indigenous elders, neuroscientists, psychiatrists, functional medicine physicians and others to seek sustainability and accessibility to people of all, regardless of race or socioeconomic status. Egos must be set aside, as well as ownership of modern molecules or plant medicines. Collaborating worldwide for ongoing respectful access, sustainability, and application of plant medicines such as Ayahuasca and Peyote through indigenous elders and shamans will be an ongoing process. Yes, this also includes slowing climate change that is threatening all plants, animals, coral reefs and our very existence. Much of this also depends on our ability to prevent the next pandemic emerging from someone's basement laboratory, or a global nuclear war, which are real and present dangers to the survival of humans, animal species, plants, and marine life.

Psychedelics offer an opportunity for us to be smarter, more creative, critical thinkers. They also encourage greater levels of empathy, love, altruism, and environmental protection. Enjoying psychedelics meditatively in the wilderness can help rewild us to our primal roots as well. Most importantly, they reconnect us to each other, nature, and the deepest states of "oneness".

New neuroplastogens are emerging from several pharmaceutical companies without the psychedelic effect (non-hallucinogenic), but with many of the benefits found in psychedelics. This is an exciting new frontier in neuroscience. As they utilize the backbone structures of plant medicines and synthetic psychedelics making them free of a psychedelic trip, they will offer a much broader therapeutic application. Especially to those who don't desire a trip-like experience, or have intolerable side effects. While it may not provide the empathogenic benefits, it may provide the neuroplastic and other benefits of psychedelics, and perhaps even more robust stimulation of BDNF. This will be applied to a select niche of patients. I will, however, remain an advocate for the classic and more affordable psychedelics that offer more transcendent benefits.

I'm hopeful that ongoing research will continue to shed light on the potential benefits of psychedelics for those on the autism spectrum. This area of exploration is especially meaningful to me, as I have a son on the spectrum. As studies evolve, I remain optimistic that these compounds may offer new avenues for treatment along with ongoing therapies. I've noticed improved emotional IQ and executive function after having him begin psychedelic therapy as an adult. Much more research is needed for those on the spectrum.

I'm also hopeful to see breakthroughs in the application of psychedelics to promote neural growth and rewiring. Perhaps combining this with stem cell therapies (Mesenchymal, Neural Stem/Progenitor Cells, Oligodendrocyte Precursor Cells, or Induced Pluripotent Stem Cells) will yield promising results.

Our world is at a tipping point. The doomsday clock is ticking towards its final seconds, as wars continue, the planet continues to warm, AI becomes a potential threat, and more pandemics and nuclear war are at our doorstep. Taking deep breaths and applying psychedelic therapies can mitigate our fears, but we must do what we can to set the clock back. I, like most of you, want a future for our children, grandchildren, and our planet. I encourage everyone to do what they can to make our world a better place.

As you've likely noticed, I've woven a thin thread of spirituality throughout this predominantly science-based content of this book. My aim isn't to sound 'woo woo,' but rather to express a truth and not hide what many will discover firsthand: when you begin working with psychedelics, you may naturally find yourself drawn toward deeper spiritual grounding and moments of profound enlightenment through your journeys.

I challenge you to find your more primal spiritual self, leaving your cell phones, laptops, and the darkness of social media behind, even if just for a weekend. Boldly walk into the wilderness with nothing but a yoga mat, a pillow, and the setting of towering trees and a blue sky above you. Enjoy your favorite psychedelic, become present in the now, and envision yourself as someone who can become stronger, smarter, less fearful, bolder, and empowered to make the world around us more loving and sustainable. As you awaken to this new potential reality of the world around you, I hope you will share your inner shamanic insights with your friends and family. In doing so, you will ripple this field of energy to heal our broken world. And if for some reason you did or did not resonate with some of this book, I'd love your feedback. Feel free to email me. I want this book to be an evolving manuscript with your help.

Above all, I wish you - and everyone on this planet - a life filled with boundless joy, vibrant health, and deep, unconditional love. May you not only discover this state of being for yourself, but also become a guiding light for others to find it, through goodwill, compassion, and perhaps even the shared wonder of psychedelic exploration...

Acknowledgement to the Pioneers of Psychedelic Medicine

I'm grateful to the Amazonian shamans, Native American shamans, Maria Sabina (Mazatec curandera-healer), and the many early pioneers of psychedelic medicine. I'd like to particularly recognize Albert Hoffman, who discovered LSD in 1938, and Alexander Shulgin, who synthesized MDMA and 2C-B. Other important more contemporary pioneers include Timothy Leary (Harvard Psychologist, LSD advocate), Richard Alpert (Guru Ram Dass), Stanislav Grof (LSD psychotherapy and holotropic breathwork) Humphry Osmand (LSD researcher and coined the term psychedelic), Rick Strassman (DMT researcher), Roland

Griffiths (psilocybin researcher), Robin Carhart-Harris (fMRI psychedelic researcher), Manish Girn (Psychedelic Researcher), David Nutt (UK psychedelic medicine research advocate), Rick Doblin (MAPS founder and MDMA advocate), James Fadiman (microdosing researcher) and Paul Stamets (mycologist, psilocybin stacking expert). To the future researchers and proponents of this movement who will carry the torch of psychedelic mindful illumination forward. Of course, to those many more I may have missed or will emerge, your work is deeply appreciated.

References

Introduction

1. *Initial Severity and Antidepressant Benefits: A Meta-Analysis of Data Submitted to the Food and Drug Administration Irving Kirsch ,Brett J Deacon,Tania B Huedo-Medina,Alan Scoboria,Thomas J Moore,Blair T Johnson Published: February 26, 2008* https://doi.org/10.1371/journal.pmed.0050045.

Chapter 1

1. Rajan KB, Weuve J, Barnes LL, McAninch EA, Wilson RS, Evans DA. Population estimate of people with clinical AD and mild cognitive impairment in the United States (2020-2060). Alzheimers Dement 2021;17(12):1966-1975.

2. "2025 Alzheimer's disease facts and figures." *Alzheimer's and Dementia*, vol. 20, no. 5, 2024, pp. 3708 - 3821, https://alz-journals.onlinelibrary.wiley.com/doi/10.1002/alz.13809.

3. "Alzheimer's Facts and Figures Report." *Alzheimer's Association*, https://www.alz.org/alzheimers-dementia/facts-figures.

4. "About Dementia | Alzheimer's Disease and Dementia." *CDC*, 17 August 2024, https://www.cdc.gov/alzheimers-dementia/about/index.html.

5. Gwira JA, Fryar CD, Gu Q. Prevalence of Total, Diagnosed, and Undiagnosed Diabetes in Adults: United States, August 2021–August 2023. 2024 Nov. In: NCHS Data Briefs [Internet]. Hyattsville (MD): National Center for Health Statistics (US); 2024 Jul-. No. 516. Available from: https://www.ncbi.nlm.nih.gov/books/NBK612760/?utm_source=chatgpt.com doi: 10.15620/cdc/165794.

6   Kilmer, B., Priest, M., et al. (2024, June 27). Magic mushrooms are the most-used psychedelic drug in the U.S.; about 3.1% of adults used Psilocybin in the past year (~8 million), and 12% reported lifetime use [Press release]. RAND Corporation.

7   Mitchell, J.M., Bogenschutz, M., Lilienstein, A. et al. MDMA-assisted therapy for severe PTSD: a randomized, double-blind, placebo-controlled phase 3 study. Nat Med 27, 1025–1033 (2021). https://doi.org/10.1038/s41591-021-01336-3.

8   Mitchell, J.M., Ot'alora G., M., van der Kolk, B. et al. MDMA-assisted therapy for moderate to severe PTSD: a randomized, placebo-controlled phase 3 trial. Nat Med 29, 2473–2480 (2023). https://doi.org/10.1038/s41591-023-02565-4.

9   https://maps.org/mdma/ptsd/phase3/

10 Banushi B, Polito V. A Comprehensive Review of the Current Status of the Cellular Neurobiology of Psychedelics. Biology (Basel). 2023 Oct 28;12(11):1380. doi: 10.3390/biology12111380. PMID: 37997979; PMCID: PMC10669348.

11 Shafiee A, Arabzadeh Bahri R, Rafiei MA, et al. The effect of psychedelics on the level of brain-derived neurotrophic factor: A systematic review and meta-analysis. Journal of Psychopharmacology. 2024;38(5):425-431. doi:10.1177/02698811241234247.

12 Pollan, Michael. *How to Change Your Mind: The New Science of Psychedelics*. Penguin Books, 2019.

13 Daws, R.E., Timmermann, C., Giribaldi, B. et al. Increased global integration in the brain after Psilocybin therapy for depression. Nat Med 28, 844–851 (2022). https://doi.org/10.1038/s41591-022-01744-z.

Chapter 2:

1   Walter Isaacson, *Steve Jobs*. Simon & Schuster 2011, Chapter 5 ("The Apple I")

2   Daws, R.E., Timmermann, C., Giribaldi, B. et al. Increased global integration in the brain after Psilocybin therapy for depression. Nat Med 28, 844–851 (2022). https://doi.org/10.1038/s41591-022-01744-z.

3   Harman, W. W., McKim, R. H., Mogar, R. E., Fadiman, J., & Stolaroff, M. J. Psychedelic Agents in Creative Problem-Solving: A Pilot Study. *Psychological Reports*, *19*(1), 211-227 (1966). https://doi.org/10.2466/pr0.1966.19.1.211

Chapter 3

1. https://www.cdc.gov/nchs/fastats/suicide.htm

2. https://www.nimh.nih.gov/health/statistics/suicide

3. U.S. Department of Veterans Affairs, Office of Suicide Prevention. 2024 National Veteran Suicide Prevention Annual Report. 2024. Retrieved July 27, 2025 from https://www.mentalhealth.va.gov/docs/data-sheets/2024/2024-Annual-Report-Part-2-of-2_508.pdf.

4. https://nebraskaexaminer.com/2024/11/11/military-veterans-are-disproportionately-affected-by-suicide-but-targeted-prevention-can-help/#:~:text=November%2011%2C%202024%205%3A00%20am&text=America's%20military%20veterans%20make%20up,veterans%20will%20die%20by%20suicide.

5. Dwivedi, Yogesh et al. "Altered gene expression of brain-derived neurotrophic factor and receptor tyrosine kinase B in postmortem brain of suicide subjects." *Archives of general psychiatry* vol. 60,8 (2003): 804-15. doi:10.1001/archpsyc.60.8.804.

6. https://www.nimh.nih.gov/health/statistics/major-depression.

7. Lee B, Wang Y, Carlson SA, et al. National, State-Level, and County-Level Prevalence Estimates of Adults Aged ≥18 Years Self-Reporting a Lifetime Diagnosis of Depression - United States, 2020. MMWR Morb Mortal Wkly Rep 2023;72:644–650. DOI: http://dx.doi.org/10.15585/mmwr.mm7224a1.

8. https://www.visualcapitalist.com/visualized-the-1s-share-of-u-s-wealth-over-time-1989-2024

9. https://www.stlouisfed.org/community-development/publications/the-state-of-us-household-wealth

10 Mitchell, J.M., Bogenschutz, M., Lilienstein, A. *et al.* MDMA-assisted therapy for severe PTSD: a randomized, double-blind, placebo-controlled phase 3 study. *Nat Med* 27, 1025–1033 (2021). https://doi.org/10.1038/s41591-021-01336-3.

11 Mitchell, J.M., Ot'alora G., M., van der Kolk, B. *et al.* MDMA-assisted therapy for moderate to severe PTSD: a randomized, placebo-controlled phase 3 trial. *Nat Med* 29, 2473–2480 (2023). https://doi.org/10.1038/s41591-023-02565-4.

12 https://maps.org/mdma/ptsd/phase3/

13 Carhart-Harris, R. L., Leech, R., Hellyer, P. J., Shanahan, M., Feilding, A., Tagliazucchi, E., ... & Nutt, D. (2014). The entropic brain: a theory of conscious states informed by neuroimaging research with psychedelic drugs. Frontiers in Human Neuroscience, 8, 20. https://doi.org/10.3389/fnhum.2014.00020

Chapter 4

1 Pollan, Michael. *How to Change Your Mind: The New Science of Psychedelics.* Penguin Books, 2019.

2 Anderson T, Petranker R, Rosenbaum D, Weissman CR, Dinh-Williams LA, Hui K, Hapke E, Farb NAS. Microdosing psychedelics: personality, mental health, and creativity differences in microdosers. Psychopharmacology (Berl). 2019 Feb;236(2):731-740. doi: 10.1007/s00213-018-5106-2. Epub 2019 Jan 2. PMID: 30604183.

3 Prochazkova, L., Lippelt, D.P., Colzato, L.S. *et al.* Exploring the effect of microdosing psychedelics on creativity in an open-label natural setting. *Psychopharmacology* 235, 3401–3413 (2018). https://doi.org/10.1007/s00213-018-5049-7.

4 Cameron, L. P., Nazarian, A., & Olson, D. E., Psychedelic Microdosing: Prevalence and Subjective Effects. *Journal of Psychoactive Drugs*, 52(2), (2020) 113–122. https://doi.org/10.1080/02791072.2020.1718250.

5 Hutten, Nadia R P W et al. "Mood and cognition after administration of low LSD doses in healthy volunteers: A placebo controlled dose-effect finding study." *European neuropsychopharmacology : the journal of the European College of Neuropsychopharmacology* vol. 41 (2020): 81-91. doi:10.1016/j.euroneuro.2020.10.002.

6 Ly, Calvin et al. "Psychedelics Promote Structural and Functional Neural Plasticity." *Cell reports* vol. 23,11 (2018): 3170-3182. doi:10.1016/j.celrep.2018.05.022.

7 Kato, K., Kleinhenz, J.M., Shin, YJ. et al. Psilocybin treatment extends cellular lifespan and improves survival of aged mice. *NPJ Aging* 11, 55 (2025). https://doi.org/10.1038/s41514-025-00244-x.

8 https://www.nccih.nih.gov/about/budget/nccih-funding-appropriations-history.

9 Alberto Fernando Oliveira Justo Regina Paradela, Natalia Gomes Goncalves, Vitor Ribeiro Paes, Renata Elaine Paraizo Leite, Ricardo Nitrini, Carlos Augusto Pasqualucci, Eduardo Ferriolli, Lea T. Grinberg and Claudia Kimie Suemoto "Association Between Alcohol Consumption, Cognitive Abilities, and Neuropathologic Changes. A Population-Based Autopsy Study". Neurology May 2025 104(9).

10 https://www.shouselaw.com/co/defense/laws/psilocybin-mushrooms/.

11 https://www.cpr.org/2023/06/21/colorado-psychedelic-law-for-psilocybin-mushrooms/.

12 https://apnews.com/article/colorado-psilocybin-psychedelic-therapy-legal-ptsd-veterans-99fc5a0703d85daa0903d5a2b2acc9be.

13 https://en.wikipedia.org/wiki/Psilocybin_decriminalization_in_the_United_States.

Chapter 5

1 https://precivityad.com/precivityad2-patients.

2 https://hopkinspsychedelic.org/alzheimers.

3 Family N, Maillet EL, Williams LT, Krediet E, Carhart-Harris RL, Williams TM, Nichols CD, Goble DJ, Raz S, "Safety, tolerability, pharmacokinetics, and pharmacodynamics of low dose lysergic acid diethylamide (LSD) in healthy older volunteers". *Psychopharmacology (Berl)*. 237 (3): 841–853 (March 2020). doi:10.1007/s00213-019-05417-7. PMC 7036065. PMID 31853557.

4 https://adisinsight.springer.com/drugs/800063629.

5   https://www.michaeljfox.org/grant/assessment-psilocybin-therapy-treatment-depression-parkinsons-disease.

6   https://parkinsonsnewstoday.com/news/psychedelic-psilocybin-clinical-trial-parkinsons-nears-end/.

7   Saeger, Hannah N, and David E Olson. "Psychedelic-inspired approaches for treating neurodegenerative disorders." *Journal of neurochemistry* vol. 162,1 (2022): 109-127. doi:10.1111/jnc.15544

8   https://en.wikipedia.org/wiki/List_of_investigational_hallucinogens_and_entactogens.

9   Szabo, Attila. "Psychedelics and Immunomodulation: Novel Approaches and Therapeutic Opportunities." *Frontiers in immunology* vol. 6 358. 14 Jul. 2015, doi:10.3389/fimmu.2015.00358.

10 https://www.politico.eu/article/eu-funds-first-psychedelic-study-in-patients-with-incurable-diseases/.

11 https://www.hopkinsmedicine.org/psychiatry/research/psychedelics-research.

12 Siegel, J.S., Subramanian, S., Perry, D. *et al.* Psilocybin desynchronizes the human brain. *Nature* 632, 131–138 (2024). https://doi.org/10.1038/s41586-024-07624-5.

13,15 https://www.pacificneuroscienceinstitute.org/blog/brain-health/ufc-fighters-brain-injury-successfully-treated-with-psychedelic-therapy/.

14 Khan M, Carter GT, Aggarwal SK and Holland J (2021) Psychedelics for Brain Injury: A Mini-Review. *Front. Neurol.* 12:685085. doi: 10.3389/fneur.2021.685085.

16 https://www.scientificamerican.com/article/this-powerful-psychedelic-shows-promise-for-relieving-traumatic-brain-injury/.

17 https://www.sciencealert.com/psilocybin-put-rat-brains-back-together-after-mild-head-trauma.

18 https://en.wikipedia.org/wiki/David_E._Olson.

19 https://www.cdc.gov/stroke/data-research/facts-stats/index.html?utm_source=chatgpt.com.

20   https://www.biospace.com/algernon-neuroscience-announces-40-patient-phase-2-psychedelic-drug-dmt-stroke-study.

21   https://psychedelichealth.co.uk/2023/01/17/first-subject-dosed-phase-1-dmt-stroke-study/.

22   https://secure.jhu.edu/form/phathom-study.

23   https://www.hopkinsmedicine.org/news/newsroom/news-releases/2023/06/study-shows-psychedelic-drugs-reopen-critical-periods-for-social-learning.

24   https://en.wikipedia.org/wiki/Dimethyltryptamine.

25   https://www.hopkinsmedicine.org/news/newsroom/news-releases/2023/06/study-shows-psychedelic-drugs-reopen-critical-periods-for-social-learning.

Chapter 6

1   Inserra, A., Giorgini, G., Lacroix, S., Bertazzo, A., Choo, J., Markopolous, A., Grant, E., Abolghasemi, A., De Gregorio, D., Flamand, N., Rogers, G., Comai, S., Silvestri, C., Gobbi, G., & Di Marzo, V. (2023). Effects of repeated lysergic acid diethylamide (LSD) on the mouse brain endocannabinoidome and gut microbiome. *British Journal of Pharmacology*, 180(6), 721–739. https://doi.org/10.1111/bph.15977.

2   https://en.wikipedia.org/wiki/Psilocybin

3   Caspani, Giorgia et al. "Mind over matter: the microbial mindscapes of psychedelics and the gut-brain axis." *Pharmacological research* vol. 207 (2024): 107338. doi:10.1016/j.phrs.2024.107338.

4   https://www.psychedelics.com/mushrooms/how-to-lemon-tek.

Chapter 7

1   Knudsen, G.M. Sustained effects of single doses of classical psychedelics in humans. *Neuropsychopharmacol*. 48, 145–150 (2023). https://doi.org/10.1038/s41386-022-01361-x.

Chapter 8

1. Erickson KI, Leckie RL, Weinstein AM. Physical activity, fitness, and gray matter volume. Neurobiol Aging. 2014 Sep;35 Suppl 2:S20-8. doi: 10.1016/j.neurobiolaging.2014.03.034. Epub 2014 May 14. PMID: 24952993; PMCID: PMC4094356.

2. Coelho-Júnior, H. J., Sampaio, R. A. C., Uchida, M. C., Teixeira, L. F. M., Caldeira, R. S. Saavedra, F. J. F., ... & Gobbi, S. Resistance Training Preserves Hippocampal Volume and White Matter Microstructure in Older Adults With Mild Cognitive Impairment: A Randomized Controlled Trial." GeroScience, 46, Article 29 (2025) https://doi.org/10.1007/s11357-024-01183-0.

3. Srámek, P et al. "Human physiological responses to immersion into water of different temperatures." *European journal of applied physiology* vol. 81,5 (2000): 436-42. doi:10.1007/s004210050065.

4. Peretti, D., Bastide, A., Radford, H. *et al.* RBM3 mediates structural plasticity and protective effects of cooling in neurodegeneration. *Nature* 518, 236–239 (2015). https://doi.org/10.1038/nature14142.

5. Agarwal P, et al. Association of Mediterranean-DASH intervention for neurodegenerative delay and Mediterranean diets with Alzheimer disease pathology. *Neurology*. 2023. Epub March 8. doi: 10.1212/wnl.0000000000207176.

6. Kirkpatrick MG, Francis SM, Lee R, de Wit H, Jacob S. Plasma oxytocin concentrations following MDMA or intranasal oxytocin in humans. Psychoneuroendocrinology. 2014 Aug;46:23-31. doi: 10.1016/j.psyneuen.2014.04.006. Epub 2014 Apr 19. PMID: 24882155; PMCID: PMC4088952.

7. https://en.wikipedia.org/wiki/Ram_Dass.

Chapter 9

1. https://www.dhs.gov/implementing-911-commission-recommendations.

2. Front. Aging Neurosci., Alzheimer's Disease and Related Dementias. Volume 15 - 2023 | https://doi.org/10.3389/fnagi.2023.1260427.

3   Davey Smith, G et al. "Sex and death: are they related? Findings from the Caerphilly Cohort Study." *BMJ (Clinical research ed.)* vol. 315,7123 (1997): 1641-4. doi:10.1136/bmj.315.7123.1641.

4   https://www.psychologytoday.com/us/blog/all-about-sex/202507/more-sex-longer-life-coincidence-or-cause-and-effect.

5   Taryn Smith, MD, NCMP and Pelin Batur, MD, FACP, NCMP "Prescribing testosterone and DHEA: The role of androgens in women"Cleveland Clinic Journal of Medicine January 2021, 88 (1) 35-43; DOI: https://doi.org/10.3949/ccjm.88a.20030.

6   http://www.thetimes.com/life-style/health-fitness/article/testosterone-for-women-ten-things-you-need-to-know-health-advice-g6wstk2c9.

7   Mengjun Zhang, Yubin Wu, Ruonan Gao, Xinwei Chen, Ruiyu Chen, Zhou Chen, Glucagon-like peptide-1 analogs mitigate neuroinflammation in Alzheimer's disease by suppressing NLRP2 activation in astrocytes,Molecular and Cellular Endocrinology, Volume 542,2022,111529, ISSN 0303-7207,https://doi.org/10.1016/j.mce.2021.111529.

8   Mingyang Sun, Xiaoling Wang, Zhongyuan Lu, Yitian Yang, Shuang Lv, Mengrong Miao, Wan-Ming Chen, Szu Yuan Wu, Jiaqiang Zhang - Evaluating GLP-1 receptor agonists versus metformin as first-line therapy for reducing dementia risk in type 2 diabetes: BMJ Open Diabetes Research & Care 2025;13:e004902.

9   https://www.alzdiscovery.org/uploads/cognitive_vitality_media/Dihexa_1.pdf.

10 Harrison DE, Strong R, Sharp ZD, Nelson JF, Astle CM, Flurkey K, Nadon NL, Wilkinson JE, Frenkel K, Carter CS, Pahor M, Javors MA, Fernandez E, Miller RA. Rapamycin fed late in life extends lifespan in genetically heterogeneous mice. Nature. 2009 Jul 16;460(7253):392-5. doi: 10.1038/nature08221. Epub 2009 Jul 8. PMID: 19587680; PMCID: PMC2786175.

11 Miller RA, Harrison DE, Astle CM, Fernandez E, Flurkey K, Han M, Javors MA, Li X, Nadon NL, Nelson JF, Pletcher S, Salmon AB, Sharp ZD, Van Roekel S, Winkleman L, Strong R. Rapamycin-mediated lifespan increase in mice is dose and sex dependent and metabolically distinct from dietary restriction. Aging Cell. 2014 Jun;13(3):468-77. doi:

10.1111/acel.12194. Epub 2014 Feb 9. PMID: 24341993; PMCID: PMC4032600.

12   Kaeberlein TL, Green AS, Haddad G, et al. Evaluation of off-label rapamycin use to promote healthspan in 333 adults. GeroScience. 2023;45(5):2757-2768. doi:10.1007/s11357-023-00818-1.

13   Caccamo A, Majumder S, Richardson A, Strong R, Oddo S. Molecular interplay between mammalian target of rapamycin (mTOR), amyloid-beta, and Tau: effects on cognitive impairments. J Biol Chem. 2010 Apr 23;285(17):13107-20. doi: 10.1074/jbc.M110.100420. Epub 2010 Feb 23. PMID: 20178983; PMCID: PMC2857107. Human trials are emerging, especially with analogs like everolimus and low-dose regimens.

14   Zhou W, et al. "Rapamycin Augments the Antidepressant Effects of Ketamine." Am J Psychiatry. 2021.

15   Hipskind SG, Grover FL Jr, Fort TR, Helffenstein D, Burke TJ, Quint SA, Bussiere G, Stone M, Hurtado T. Pulsed Transcranial Red/Near-Infrared Light Therapy Using Light-Emitting Diodes Improves Cerebral Blood Flow and Cognitive Function in Veterans with Chronic Traumatic Brain Injury: A Case Series. Photobiomodul Photomed Laser Surg. 2019 Feb;37(2):77-84. doi: 10.1089/photob.2018.4489. PMID: 31050928; PMCID: PMC6390875.

16   Aron, L., Ngian, Z.K., Qiu, C. et al. Lithium deficiency and the onset of Alzheimer's disease. Nature (2025). https://doi.org/10.1038/s41586-025-09335-x

17   Gonzalez-Lima, F, and Allison Auchter. "Protection against neurodegeneration with low-dose methylene blue and near-infrared light." *Frontiers in cellular neuroscience* vol. 9 179. 12 May. 2015, doi:10.3389/fncel.2015.00179.

18   Wang Aoao , Ma Xinbo , Bian Jiaqi , Jiao Zhenrui , Zhu Qiuyi , Wang Peng , Zhao Yantao. Signalling pathways underlying pulsed electromagnetic fields in bone repair. Frontiers in Bioengineering and Biotechnology Volume 12 - 2024.

19   Dedoncker, J., Brunoni, A. R., Baeken, C., & Vanderhasselt, MA. A systematic review and meta-analysis of the effects of transcranial direct current stimulation (tDCS) over the dorsolateral prefrontal cor-

tex in healthy and neuropsychiatric samples: Influence of stimulation parameters. Brain Stimulation, 9(4), 501–517 2016. https://doi.org/10.1016/j.brs.2016.04.006.

20. Chen Liang , Xiong Ye , Chopp Michael , Zhang Yanlu Engineered exosomes enriched with select microRNAs amplify their therapeutic efficacy for traumatic brain injury and stroke. Frontiers in Cellular Neuroscience. Volume 18 - 2024.

20. Regmi Shobha, Liu Daniel Dan, Shen Michelle, Kevadiya Bhavesh D., Ganguly Abantika, Primavera Rosita, Chetty Shashank, Yarani Reza, Thakor Avnesh S. Mesenchymal stromal cells for the treatment of Alzheimer's disease: Strategies and limitations.Frontiers in Molecular Neuroscience.Volume 15 - 2022.

Image References

1. 5HT2A and Serotonin Receptor

2. NMDA Antagonist

3. BDNF Stimulation Chart

    Supporting references for chart generation include :Ly et al., Cell Reports (2018): "LSD promotes structural and functional neural plasticity through 5-HT2A receptor activation." https://doi.org/10.1016/j.celrep.2018.05.022, Catlow et al., Experimental Brain Research (2013): "Psilocybin facilitates hippocampal neurogenesis and extinction of fear memory." https://doi.org/10.1007/s00221-013-3530-7, Dakic et al., Frontiers in Neuroscience (2017): "Short term changes in the proteome of human cerebral organoids induced by 5-MeO-DMT." https://doi.org/10.3389/fnins.2017.00523, Szabo et al., Neuropsychopharmacology (2016): "The potent sigma-1 receptor agonist 5-MeO-DMT enhances neurogenesis and plasticity." https://doi.org/10.1038/npp.2016.78, Morales-García et al., Translational Psychiatry (2020): "Ayahuasca stimulates BDNF expression and adult neurogenesis. https://doi.org/10.1038/s41398-020-0703-3, Marton et al., PLOS ONE (2019): "Ibogaine stimulates BDNF and GDNF expression in the rat brain." https://doi.org/10.1371/journal.pone.0211028, Duman & Aghajanian, Science (2012): "Synaptic dysfunction in depression: potential therapeutic targets." https://doi.org/10.1126/science.1222939, Young et al., Biological Psychiatry (2014): "MDMA increases BDNF in the hippocampus of rats."https://doi.org/10.1016/j.biopsych.2014.06.010,

    Kivell et al., Frontiers in Pharmacology (2014): "Salvinorin A: psychoactive kappa-opioid effects without clear BDNF upregulation." https://doi.org/10.3389/fphar.2014.00050.

4. Anatomy of a Neuron and Synapse (Shutterstock 2445508897)

5. Default Mode Network (Wikipedia)

6. fMRI before and after LSD. Credit: Imperial College of London. https://www.imperial.ac.uk/news/171699/the-brain-lsd-revealed-first-scans/

7. Functional Brain Network Communication. Petri et al./Proceedings of the Royal Society Interface. 2014 Dec 6;11(101):20140873.

8. Ammonites and Fibonacci Sequence. (Author photo and Shutterstock 1670795137)

9. Relative Harm Chart- by David Nutt

10. Dendritic Spines (Wikipedia)

11. Ayahuasca Brew, vine, and Chacruna (Shutterstock 1131880895)

12. Impact of Prolonged Stress influencing Glucose Metabolism

13. Pumping Iron can Pump your Brain!

14. Being in Flow with nature (Shutterstock 31193010)

15. Fractal Geometry in Brain Coral (Shutterstock 2440546943)

16. Hugs can increase oxytocin

17. The impact of sleep apnea on the Brain

18. Dr. Grover's Regenerative Medicine Algorhythm

19. GLP-1 Benefits

20. Basic Mitochondrial Structure(Shutterstock 2545082157)

21. NAD+ Synthesis (Shutterstock 2296669835)

Recommended Reading

Pollan, Michael. *How to Change Your Mind: What the New Science of Psychedelics Teaches Us About Consciousness, Dying, Addiction, Depression, and Transcendence.* Penguin Press, 2018.

Nutt, David. (2023).Psychedelics: The Revolutionary Drugs That Could Change Your Life – A Guide from the Expert. London: Yellow Kite (an imprint of Hodder & Stoughton).

Fadiman, J. (2011). The Psychedelic Explorer's Guide: Safe, Therapeutic, and Sacred Journeys. Rochester, VT: Park Street Press.

Carhart-Harris, Robin, Upcoming book in Fall 2025: "How Psychedelics Work: Illuminating the Hidden Mind".

Bredesen, Dale E. *The End of Alzheimer's: The First Program to Prevent and Reverse Cognitive Decline.* Avery, 2017.

Bredesen, Dale E. The Ageless Brain: How to sharpen and protect your mind for a lifetime. Flatiron Books, 2025.

Perlmutter, David & Colman, Carol The Better Brain Book: The best tool for improving memory and sharpness and preventing aging of the brain. Penguin Publishing 2005.

Stamets, Paul, ed. Fantastic Fungi: How Mushrooms Can Heal, Shift Consciousness, and Save the Planet. San Rafael, CA: Earth Aware Editions, 2019.

Stamets, Paul. Psilocybin Mushrooms in Their Natural Habitats: A Guide to the History, Identification, and Use of Psychoactive Fungi. Ten Speed Press. 2025.

Grof, Stanislav & Grof, Christina. Holotropic Breathwork, Second Edition: A New Approach to Self-Exploration and Therapy. Albany, NY: State University of New York (SUNY) Press 2023.

Strassman, Rick. DMT: The Spirit Molecule: A Doctor's Revolutionary Research into the Biology of Near-Death and Mystical Experiences. Park Street Press, 2001.

Grey, Alex. Net of Being. Inner Traditions, 2012. and his 2024 Entheon Museum book.

Shulgin, Alexander, and Ann Shulgin. TIHKAL: The Continuation. Transform Press, 1997.

Shulgin, Alexander, and Ann Shulgin. PIHKAL: A Chemical Love Story. Transform Press, 1991.

Tolle, Eckhart. *The Power of Now: A Guide to Spiritual Enlightenment*. New World Library, 1997.

Tolle, Eckhart. 2005. *A New Earth: Awakening to Your Life's Purpose*. New York: Dutton/Penguin.

Dass, Ram. Be Here Now. Lama Foundation, 1971.

McKenna, Terence. Food of the Gods: The Search for the Original Tree of Knowledge. Bantam Books, 1992.

Huxley, Aldous. The Doors of Perception. Harper & Brothers, 1954.

Villoldo, Alberto. Shaman, Healer, Sage: How to Heal Yourself and Others with the Energy Medicine of the Americas. Harmony Books, 2000.

Grover, Fred. Spiritual Genomics: A Physician's Deep Dive Beyond Conventional Medicine to Discover Unique Keys to Your Healing, Longevity and Personal Evolution. 2016.

Recommended Websites

- **MAPS** (Multidisciplinary Association for Psychedelic Studies) https://maps.org

- **Johns Hopkins** Center for Psychedelic and Consciousness Research https://hopkinspsychedelic.org

- **Imperial College London** Centre for Psychedelic Research https://www.imperial.ac.uk/psychedelic-research-centre

- **Psychedelic Scientist**-Manish Girn PhD. https://maneshgirn.com/the-psychedelic-scientist/

About the Author

Fred Grover Jr. M.D. is a Family Physician who specializes in preventative, functional, regenerative, and psychedelic medicine in Denver, Colorado. He graduated from the University of Louisville School of Medicine, and completed his residency at the University of Colorado Family Medicinte Program where he was Chief Resident, and was awarded the Colorado Family Medicine Resident of the Year in 1996. He has continued to teach medical students in his private practice in Integrative Medicine electives, and has been active in volunteer medical work in Nepal in the past. He has also volunteered his time toward public health initiatives and legislation to reduce harm from tobacco and guns, and has helped promote the decriminalization of psilocybin and other psychedelics. He is an adventurer and lover of the outdoors who enjoys hiking, paddling, sailing, scuba diving, skiing and other activities with family and friends. His mindful based activities, particularly in shamanic circles abroad, have helped him stay centered in this chaotic world, while opening his mind to finding better solutions for planetary sustainability. In addition to being an avid reader, he has written two other books; Spiritual Genomics, and Awakening Gaia. Visit FredGroverMD.com to learn more about him.

About the Cover Artist, Martin Bridges

Martin Bridge is an animist, artist, and educator who lives and creates in the hills of western Massachusetts. One of the most central themes to his work is an exploration of the natural world and our place as humans in relation to the web of life that we are a part of. His work bridges realms of science and mysticism in an effort to challenge the cultural paradigms that dictate how we relate to both the natural world as well as our brothers and sisters. As an avid Permaculture designer and mycologist he strives to create work that improves his own awareness of how we relate to nature and invites viewers to contemplate the same.

Martin has been a driving force in psychedelic advocacy in New England working with local legislators and supporting groups that are advancing initiatives in Maine and Massachusetts including Mass Healing and the Northeast Alliance for Psychedelic Access. Among the myriad of reasons he feels called to advance Psychedelic medicines is the quality of "Nature Empathy" that many instill. As in his own experience, the visceral sense of interconnectedness many feel inspires a greater calling to defend the web of life and adopt regenerative practices. Through his work he hopes to inspire and cultivate a greater sense of mystery and possibility in our experience of the world. His creative design of the beautiful cover is much appreciated! Check out his work at: https://thebridgebrothers.com/artist/martin-bridge/

www.ingramcontent.com/pod-product-compliance
Lightning Source LLC
Chambersburg PA
CBHW051543020426
42333CB00016B/2075